PEPTIC ULCER DIET COOKBOOK FOR BEGINNERS

100+ Nourishing Anti-Inflammatory Recipes for Soothing Ulcer Symptoms and Enhancing Digestive Health

Kingsley Klopp

To show our appreciation for your purchase, we're delighted to offer you these special bonuses as a heartfelt thank you.

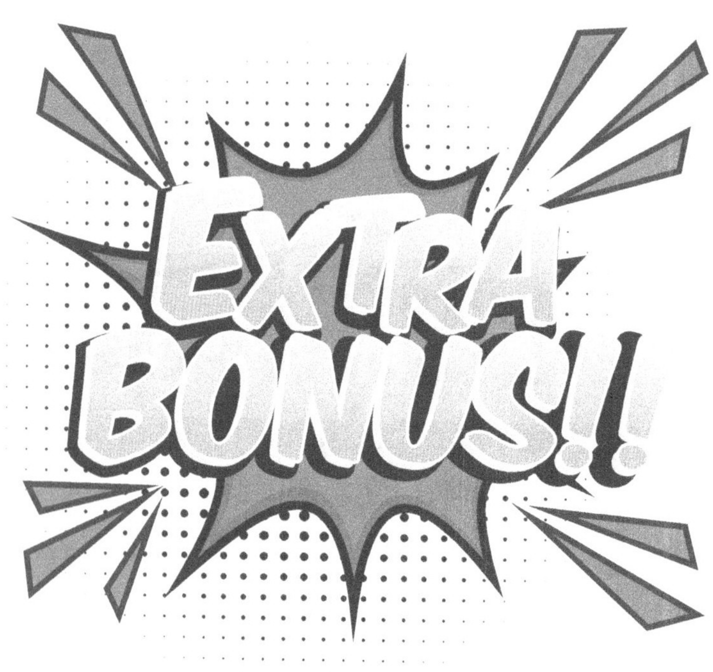

1. A Food Tracker Journal
2. Downloadable E-BOOK featuring full-color images of finished recipes

Table of Contents

Vegetables

Important Note

We understand that living with peptic ulcers can be challenging, impacting your daily life and dietary choices. This cookbook is designed to provide you with delicious meal options that are gentle on your stomach while promoting healing and well-being.

It's important to note that individual dietary needs vary. While the recipes in this cookbook are crafted with sensitivity to peptic ulcers, we encourage you to adjust them according to your personal preferences and health requirements. Consulting with your healthcare provider or a registered dietitian is recommended, especially if you have questions or uncertainties about how to integrate these recipes into your diet. They can offer personalized guidance to ensure that the foods you choose support your overall treatment plan.

Please be aware that the nutritional information provided with each recipe is approximate. Factors such as ingredient variations, portion sizes, and cooking methods can impact the final nutritional content of your meals. Use this information as a general guideline and consider it alongside professional advice for a well-rounded understanding of your dietary intake.

Furthermore, If our cookbook has brought joy to your kitchen and table, we'd be thrilled to hear about your experiences in an Amazon review. On the flip side, if you stumble upon any hiccups while exploring our recipes, don't hesitate to get in touch at **kloppkingsley@gmail.com.** We're here to support your cooking journey every step of the way.

As you explore the recipes in this cookbook, we encourage you to approach them with curiosity and creativity. Discover new flavors, experiment with wholesome ingredients, and enjoy the process of nourishing yourself with meals that support your digestive health and overall wellness.

Introduction

Hey there! Ever had that burning sensation in your stomach that just won't go away? Maybe it feels like there's a fire brewing inside after you eat, leaving you uncomfortable and unsure about what foods to trust. If you've been diagnosed with a peptic ulcer, you know exactly what I'm talking about. But here's the thing: managing your diet doesn't have to be a mystery or a source of stress. Welcome to the **Peptic Ulcer Diet Cookbook for Beginners,** your go-to guide for delicious meals that won't aggravate your stomach but will still make your taste buds sing.

Living with a peptic ulcer means walking a tightrope with every meal. You want to eat to nourish your body, but you also want to avoid triggering that uncomfortable burning sensation. It's a delicate balance, but this cookbook is here to help you navigate it with confidence. We've packed it with easy-to-follow recipes that are not only gentle on your stomach but also packed with flavor. Think of it as your roadmap to enjoying food again, without the fear of discomfort. Cooking for a peptic ulcer isn't just about what you can't eat; it's about discovering what you can. That's where our cookbook shines. From soothing soups and comforting stews to light, refreshing salads and satisfying main dishes, each recipe is carefully crafted to be stomach-friendly while still satisfying your cravings. We've taken the guesswork out of meal planning so you can focus on enjoying your food and feeling good afterward. We get it—changing your diet can feel daunting, especially when you're already dealing with health challenges. But rest assured, you're not alone on this journey. This cookbook is designed specifically with beginners in mind, whether you're just starting to explore the kitchen or looking for new ways to adapt your favorite meals to fit your dietary needs. We'll walk you through everything, step by step, so you can feel confident and empowered in your culinary skills.

Beyond just recipes, we're here to educate and empower you. Understanding how different foods affect your stomach can make a world of difference in managing your peptic ulcer. That's why we provide practical tips and insights throughout the book, helping you make informed choices about what to eat and why. Knowledge is power, and with the right information at your fingertips, you'll be better equipped to take control of your diet and your health. Let's talk about taste. Just because you're eating for your health doesn't mean you have to sacrifice flavor. Our recipes are designed to be both nutritious and delicious, proving that eating well can be a pleasure, not a chore. Whether you're whipping up a quick breakfast, preparing a hearty dinner for family and friends, or treating yourself to a nutritious snack, we've got you covered with recipes that are sure to satisfy.

Of course, we understand that everyone's journey with a peptic ulcer is different. What works for one person may not work for another, and that's okay. That's why this cookbook encourages flexibility and experimentation. Feel free to tweak recipes to suit your tastes and dietary needs. And if you ever feel uncertain or need personalized advice, don't hesitate to reach out to your healthcare provider. They're there to support you on your path to wellness.

As you dive into the **Peptic Ulcer Diet Cookbook for Beginners,** think of it as more than just a collection of recipes. It's your partner in health, your guide to eating well, and your ticket to reclaiming the joy of food. Cooking should be enjoyable and nourishing, and we're excited to embark on this culinary adventure with you. Together, let's discover the delicious possibilities that await in every chapter. So, grab your apron, sharpen your knives, and get ready to cook your way to a healthier, happier you. Here's to good food, good health, and a new chapter of culinary exploration!

Part 1

Understanding Peptic Ulcers
What is a Peptic Ulcer?

A peptic ulcer is a sore that forms on the lining of the stomach, small intestine, or esophagus. It can be an excruciatingly painful condition that significantly affects one's quality of life. Imagine the feeling of a relentless, burning sensation in your stomach, coupled with nausea and a gnawing hunger pang even when you've just eaten. This is the daily reality for many individuals suffering from peptic ulcers. The history of peptic ulcers is as old as humanity itself. Ancient civilizations recorded cases of what we now know as peptic ulcers, describing symptoms that resemble the condition in texts dating back thousands of years. For centuries, the cause of these ulcers was a mystery. Early medical practitioners often attributed them to stress, spicy foods, or an overabundance of stomach acid. These theories, though partially correct, did not capture the full picture.

The journey to understanding peptic ulcers took a significant turn in the early 19th century. Dr. William Beaumont, an American army surgeon, conducted groundbreaking research on the digestive system. His studies on a patient with a gastric fistula allowed him to observe the stomach's inner workings firsthand. Beaumont's work laid the foundation for modern gastroenterology, providing valuable insights into how the stomach produces acid and digests food. Despite these advancements, the true cause of peptic ulcers remained elusive until the late 20th century. In the 1980s, two Australian scientists, Dr. Barry Marshall and Dr. Robin Warren, made a discovery that revolutionized our understanding of peptic ulcers. They identified a spiral-shaped bacterium, Helicobacter pylori (H. pylori), as a major contributor to the development of peptic ulcers. This discovery was initially met with skepticism, as the prevailing belief held that no bacteria could survive in the acidic environment of the stomach. Marshall and Warren's persistence paid off when they successfully demonstrated that H. pylori infection could cause gastritis and peptic ulcers. Their groundbreaking work earned them the Nobel Prize in Physiology or Medicine in 2005. This discovery not only changed the way peptic ulcers were treated but also saved countless lives by shifting the focus from solely managing symptoms to eradicating the underlying infection.

Treatment of peptic ulcers has evolved significantly over the years. Before the discovery of H. pylori, treatment primarily involved lifestyle changes, dietary modifications, and medications to reduce stomach acid. While these methods provided some relief, they did not address the root cause of the ulcers. With the recognition of H. pylori's role, antibiotics became a crucial component of treatment, effectively curing many patients and reducing the recurrence of ulcers.

Another significant development in the treatment of peptic ulcers was the introduction of proton pump inhibitors (PPIs) and H2-receptor antagonists. These medications work by reducing the production of stomach acid, allowing the ulcer to heal and preventing further damage. Combined with antibiotics to eradicate H. pylori, these treatments have made peptic ulcers a much more manageable condition. The story of peptic ulcers is not just one of scientific discovery but also of human resilience. Living with a peptic ulcer can be a daunting experience. The constant pain and discomfort can make even the simplest tasks feel overwhelming. Yet, many people with peptic ulcers find ways to adapt and persevere, drawing on their inner strength and the support of loved ones.

Diet and lifestyle play a crucial role in managing peptic ulcers. While we now understand that H. pylori is a primary cause, factors like stress, smoking, and certain medications can exacerbate the condition. Patients are often advised to avoid foods and beverages that can irritate the stomach lining, such as spicy foods, caffeine, and alcohol. Instead, a diet rich in fruits, vegetables, and lean proteins is recommended to support healing and overall health. Living with a peptic ulcer requires a delicate balance. It means listening to your body, recognizing the signs of distress, and taking proactive steps to mitigate pain. It means finding solace in the small victories, like a day without pain or a night of restful sleep. It also means staying informed and working closely with healthcare providers to ensure the best possible outcomes.

In summary, a peptic ulcer is more than just a physical ailment; it is a testament to the complexities of the human body and the remarkable strides of medical science. From ancient misconceptions to modern breakthroughs, the journey of understanding and treating peptic ulcers is a story of discovery, perseverance, and hope. As we continue to learn more about this condition, we move closer to a future where peptic ulcers can be effectively managed, allowing individuals to lead healthier, happier lives.

Causes and Risk Factors of Peptic Ulcers

Causes

1. **Helicobacter pylori (H. pylori) Infection:**
   - Primary Cause: The most common cause of peptic ulcers is an infection with the bacterium Helicobacter pylori. This spiral-shaped bacterium thrives in the acidic environment of the stomach. It weakens the stomach's mucous lining, making it more susceptible to damage from stomach acid. The infection can lead to chronic inflammation (gastritis) and, eventually, ulcer formation.
   - Transmission: H. pylori is typically acquired during childhood through person-to-person contact, such as through saliva, vomit, or fecal matter. It can also be transmitted through contaminated food or water.
2. **Nonsteroidal Anti-Inflammatory Drugs (NSAIDs):**
   - Medications: Regular use of NSAIDs, such as aspirin, ibuprofen, and naproxen, is a significant cause of peptic ulcers. These drugs inhibit the production of prostaglandins, substances that help protect the stomach lining from the corrosive effects of stomach acid. Without adequate prostaglandins, the mucous layer is compromised, increasing the risk of ulcer formation.
   - Vulnerability: The risk is higher for individuals who take high doses of NSAIDs, use them for extended periods, or have a history of ulcer disease.
3. **Excess Stomach Acid:**
   - Hyperacidity: Conditions that cause the stomach to produce excessive acid can lead to peptic ulcers. Zollinger-Ellison syndrome, a rare condition in which tumors in the pancreas or duodenum cause overproduction of stomach acid, is an example. Excess acid can overwhelm the protective mechanisms of the stomach lining, leading to ulceration.
4. **Smoking:**
   - Tobacco Use: Smoking increases the risk of developing peptic ulcers and slows the healing of existing ones. Nicotine stimulates the stomach to produce more acid and reduces the production of bicarbonate, which neutralizes acid. Smoking also impairs blood flow to the stomach lining, hindering the healing process.
5. **Alcohol Consumption:**
   - Irritation and Damage: Excessive alcohol intake can irritate and erode the mucous lining of the stomach and increase stomach acid production. Chronic alcohol use can significantly elevate the risk of peptic ulcers and complicate their treatment.

6. Other Infections:

- Viral and Fungal Infections: Although less common, other infections such as those caused by the cytomegalovirus (CMV) or fungi in immunocompromised individuals can contribute to peptic ulcer development.

Risk Factors

1. **Age:**
   - Older Adults: The risk of peptic ulcers increases with age. Older adults are more likely to use NSAIDs, have H. pylori infections, and suffer from other health conditions that affect the stomach lining.
2. **Genetics:**
   - Family History: A family history of peptic ulcers can increase an individual's risk, suggesting a genetic predisposition to the condition. Certain genetic factors may make some people more susceptible to H. pylori infection or the damaging effects of stomach acid.
3. **Stress:**
   - Psychological Stress: While stress alone does not cause peptic ulcers, it can exacerbate symptoms and slow the healing process. Stress may lead to behaviors that increase ulcer risk, such as smoking, alcohol consumption, and the use of NSAIDs.
4. **Diet:**
   - Spicy and Acidic Foods: Although diet alone is not a direct cause of peptic ulcers, consuming foods that irritate the stomach lining, such as spicy or acidic foods, can aggravate symptoms and contribute to discomfort.
5. **Other Medical Conditions:**
   - Chronic Illnesses: Individuals with chronic illnesses, such as liver disease, kidney disease, or chronic obstructive pulmonary disease (COPD), may have an increased risk of developing peptic ulcers. These conditions can affect overall health and the body's ability to repair the stomach lining.
6. **Medications and Treatments:**
   - Corticosteroids and Blood Thinners: The use of corticosteroids and blood thinners, particularly in combination with NSAIDs, can significantly increase the risk of peptic ulcers. These medications can weaken the stomach lining and impair its ability to heal.
7. **Environmental Factors:**
   - Living Conditions: In developing countries, where H. pylori infection is more prevalent due to poor sanitation and crowded living conditions, the risk of peptic ulcers is higher. Improved hygiene and living conditions have contributed to a decline in H. pylori-related ulcers in developed countries.

Symptoms and Diagnosis of Peptic Ulcers

Symptoms
1. **Burning Stomach Pain:**
   - Description: The most common symptom of a peptic ulcer is a burning or gnawing pain in the stomach area. This pain often occurs between meals and at night when the stomach is empty. It can last from a few minutes to several hours.
   - Location: The pain is typically located in the upper abdomen, but it can also be felt in the back.
   - Relief: Eating food or taking antacids can temporarily relieve the pain, as they neutralize stomach acid or coat the ulcer.
2. **Bloating and Belching:**
   - Discomfort: Many individuals with peptic ulcers experience a feeling of fullness or bloating, which can be uncomfortable. Belching frequently is another common symptom, which may provide temporary relief from the bloating.
3. **Indigestion:**
   - Dyspepsia: Indigestion, or dyspepsia, is a frequent symptom of peptic ulcers. It can include nausea, a sense of heaviness or discomfort in the stomach, and a feeling of fullness after eating small amounts of food.
4. Heartburn:
   - Acid Reflux: Heartburn, characterized by a burning sensation in the chest, can occur when stomach acid flows back into the esophagus. This is common in individuals with peptic ulcers, particularly when lying down or after meals.
5. **Nausea and Vomiting:**
   - Digestive Distress: Nausea is a common symptom, and in some cases, it may lead to vomiting. Vomiting can be a sign of a more severe ulcer or complication, especially if it contains blood or resembles coffee grounds, indicating digested blood.
6. **Loss of Appetite and Weight Loss:**
   - Reduced Intake: Due to the discomfort associated with eating, many individuals with peptic ulcers may experience a loss of appetite. This can lead to unintended weight loss over time.
7. **Bloody or Dark Stools:**
   - Internal Bleeding: One of the more alarming symptoms of a peptic ulcer is the presence of blood in the stool. Stools may appear black or tarry due to digested blood, which indicates bleeding in the stomach or upper intestines. This is a sign of a serious complication and requires immediate medical attention.

8. Anemia:
- Fatigue and Weakness: Chronic blood loss from a bleeding ulcer can lead to anemia, which is characterized by fatigue, weakness, and pallor. Anemia occurs when there aren't enough red blood cells to carry adequate oxygen to the body's tissues.

Diagnosis

Diagnosing a peptic ulcer involves a thorough evaluation by a healthcare provider. The process typically includes the following steps:

1. **Medical History and Physical Examination:**
   - Patient Interview: The healthcare provider will start by taking a detailed medical history, asking about the patient's symptoms, lifestyle, and any medications they are taking, particularly NSAIDs.
   - Physical Examination: During the physical examination, the doctor may palpate the abdomen to check for tenderness or pain, which can indicate an ulcer.
2. **Laboratory Tests:**
   - Blood Tests: Blood tests can help detect anemia caused by a bleeding ulcer and may be used to check for the presence of H. pylori antibodies.
   - Stool Tests: A stool sample may be tested for the presence of blood or H. pylori antigens.
3. **Non-Invasive Tests for H. pylori:**
   - Urea Breath Test: This test involves swallowing a urea solution labeled with a special carbon atom. If H. pylori is present, the bacteria will break down the urea, releasing carbon dioxide that can be detected in the breath.
   - Stool Antigen Test: This test detects H. pylori proteins in a stool sample.
4. **Endoscopy:**
   - Procedure: Upper gastrointestinal endoscopy (esophagogastroduodenoscopy or EGD) is a common procedure used to diagnose peptic ulcers. A flexible tube with a camera (endoscope) is inserted through the mouth and down into the stomach and duodenum.
   - Visual Examination: The doctor can directly visualize the ulcer and may take biopsies to check for H. pylori infection or rule out cancer.
5. **Imaging Tests:**
   - Barium Swallow: For patients who cannot undergo endoscopy, a barium swallow (upper GI series) may be used. The patient drinks a barium solution that coats the lining of the esophagus, stomach, and duodenum. X-rays are then taken to identify ulcers.
6. **Biopsy:**
   - Sample Analysis: During an endoscopy, the doctor may take small tissue samples (biopsies) from the ulcer site. These samples are examined under a microscope to check for cancer cells and H. pylori infection.

The Role of Diet in Managing Peptic Ulcers

The diagnosis of a peptic ulcer can be a daunting and overwhelming experience. The persistent pain, discomfort, and worry about eating the wrong foods can turn mealtime into a stressful ordeal. However, the power of diet in managing peptic ulcers is profound, offering a beacon of hope and relief. The right dietary choices can not only soothe symptoms but also promote healing and prevent recurrence, transforming the way individuals live with this condition.

Healing Foods and Their Impact

1. **Fiber-Rich Foods:**
   - Soothing and Protective: High-fiber foods like fruits, vegetables, and whole grains are gentle on the stomach and aid in digestion. They create a protective layer on the stomach lining, reducing the irritation caused by stomach acid. Incorporating foods like oatmeal, apples, and carrots can provide a calming effect, making meals more enjoyable and less painful.
   - Emotional Relief: Eating fiber-rich foods can bring a sense of normalcy and comfort. Knowing that these foods are not only safe but beneficial, individuals can enjoy their meals without the constant fear of triggering ulcer pain.

2. **Probiotic-Rich Foods:**
   - Gut Health Enhancers: Probiotics found in yogurt, kefir, and fermented foods like sauerkraut and kimchi help maintain a healthy balance of stomach bacteria. They can combat the harmful effects of H. pylori, the bacterium responsible for many peptic ulcers, by promoting the growth of beneficial bacteria.
   - Hope and Healing: Including probiotics in the diet can instill a sense of proactive healing. The idea that every spoonful of yogurt or sip of kefir is fighting the ulcer from within can be incredibly empowering.

3. **Lean Proteins:**
   - Gentle Nourishment: Lean proteins such as chicken, turkey, tofu, and fish are less likely to irritate the stomach compared to fatty or fried meats. These proteins provide essential nutrients needed for tissue repair and overall health.
   - Comfort in Simplicity: Simple, well-cooked lean proteins can become comfort foods. They are easy to prepare and digest, offering a reliable source of nutrition that doesn't aggravate the ulcer.

4. Non-Acidic Vegetables and Fruits:
- Anti-Inflammatory Benefits: Vegetables like broccoli, spinach, and kale, and non-acidic fruits such as bananas, melons, and pears, are excellent choices. They are packed with vitamins and minerals that support healing and reduce inflammation.
- Joy of Eating: Being able to enjoy a colorful salad or a sweet, ripe melon without pain brings back the joy of eating. It transforms meals from a source of anxiety to moments of pleasure and nourishment.

5. Healthy Fats:
- Stomach-Friendly Options: Healthy fats like those found in avocados, olive oil, and nuts are beneficial. They provide essential fatty acids that aid in the repair of the stomach lining without triggering acid overproduction.
- Balanced Satisfaction: Adding a drizzle of olive oil to a salad or a handful of nuts to a snack can add flavor and satisfaction, making meals more enjoyable and varied.

Foods to Avoid and Why

1. **Spicy and Acidic Foods:**
   - Irritants: Spicy foods, citrus fruits, tomatoes, and vinegar can exacerbate ulcer pain and cause irritation. They increase stomach acid production and can inflame the stomach lining.
   - Fear of Flare-Ups: Avoiding these foods is crucial, as their consumption often leads to a painful reminder of the condition. Eliminating these irritants can reduce the fear and anxiety associated with eating.

2. **Caffeinated and Carbonated Beverages:**
   - Acid Stimulators: Coffee, tea, sodas, and energy drinks can increase stomach acid production, leading to discomfort and pain. Carbonation can cause bloating and pressure, adding to the distress.
   - Peace of Mind: Cutting out these beverages can bring a sense of peace, knowing that each drink is one step closer to a pain-free life. Opting for herbal teas and water provides hydration without the risk of discomfort.

3. **Alcohol:**
   - Harmful Effects: Alcohol irritates the stomach lining and increases acid production, which can worsen ulcers and delay healing. It can also interfere with medications prescribed for ulcer treatment.
   - Healthy Choices: Abstaining from alcohol can lead to clearer thinking and healthier decisions. Replacing alcohol with soothing alternatives like chamomile tea can provide comfort and promote healing.

4. Fatty and Fried Foods:
- Difficult to Digest: High-fat and fried foods slow down digestion and increase the risk of acid reflux, which can aggravate ulcer symptoms.
- Simple Pleasures: Avoiding these foods encourages simpler, more wholesome eating habits. Grilled or baked options can be equally satisfying without the associated risks.

Breakfast Recipes

1. Soft French Toast

Ingredients:

- 4 slices of whole-grain bread
- 2 large eggs
- 1/2 cup of low-fat milk
- 1 teaspoon of vanilla extract
- 1/2 teaspoon of ground cinnamon
- 1 tablespoon of unsalted butter
- 1 tablespoon of honey or maple syrup (optional, for serving)
- Fresh berries (optional, for serving)

Instructions:

1. In a medium bowl, whisk together the eggs, milk, vanilla extract, and ground cinnamon until well combined.
2. Dip each slice of bread into the egg mixture, ensuring both sides are well-coated.
3. In a large non-stick skillet, melt the butter over medium heat.
4. Place the coated bread slices in the skillet and cook for 2-3 minutes on each side, or until golden brown and cooked through.
5. Remove from the skillet and serve immediately with a drizzle of honey or maple syrup and fresh berries, if desired.

Nutrition Info (Per Serving):

- Calories: 250
- Protein: 10g
- Carbohydrates: 30g
- Dietary Fiber: 4g
- Sugars: 10g
- Total Fat: 10g
- Saturated Fat: 4g
- Sodium: 200mg

Serves:

- **2 servings (2 slices per serving)**

Cooking Time:

- **Total: 10 minutes**

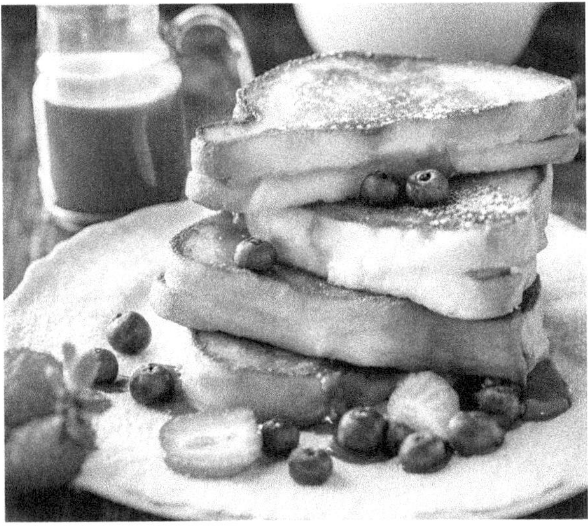

2. Puffed Rice with Milk

Ingredients:

- 2 cups of puffed rice cereal
- 1 cup of low-fat milk (or plant-based milk such as almond or oat milk)
- 1 teaspoon of honey or maple syrup
- 1/4 cup of sliced banana
- 1/4 cup of blueberries

Instructions:

1. Pour the puffed rice cereal into a bowl.
2. Heat the milk in a small saucepan over low heat until warm, but not boiling.
3. Pour the warm milk over the puffed rice cereal.
4. Drizzle with honey or maple syrup.
5. Top with sliced banana and blueberries.
6. Serve immediately.

Nutrition Info (Per Serving):

- Calories: 180
- Protein: 6g
- Carbohydrates: 35g
- Dietary Fiber: 3g
- Sugars: 15g
- Total Fat: 3g
- Saturated Fat: 1g
- Sodium: 90mg

Serves:

- 2 servings

Cooking Time:

- **Total: 5 minutes**

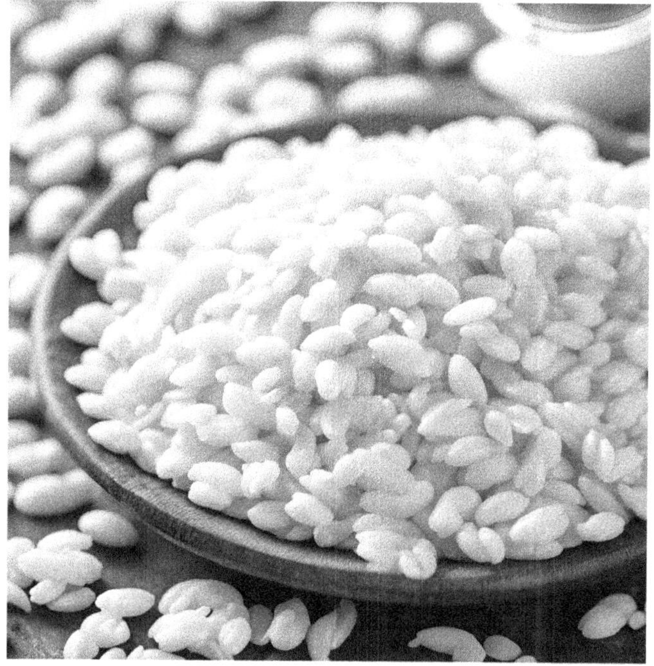

3. Sweet Potato and Kale Hash

Ingredients:

- 2 medium sweet potatoes, peeled and diced
- 2 tablespoons of olive oil
- 1 cup of chopped kale (stems removed)
- 1/2 teaspoon of ground cumin
- 1/2 teaspoon of paprika
- 2 large eggs
- 1/4 cup of shredded low-fat cheese (optional)
- Fresh parsley for garnish

Instructions:

1. In a large skillet, heat the olive oil over medium heat.
2. Add the diced sweet potatoes to the skillet and cook for about 10-12 minutes, stirring occasionally, until they are tender and slightly crispy.
3. Add the chopped kale to the skillet and cook for another 3-4 minutes, until the kale is wilted.
4. Sprinkle the ground cumin and paprika over the sweet potato and kale mixture, stirring to combine.
5. Create two small wells in the sweet potato and kale mixture and crack an egg into each well.
6. Cover the skillet and cook for about 4-5 minutes, or until the eggs are cooked to your desired doneness.
7. If using, sprinkle shredded low-fat cheese over the hash during the last minute of cooking.
8. Garnish with fresh parsley before serving.

Nutrition Info (Per Serving):

- Calories: 350
- Protein: 12g
- Carbohydrates: 45g
- Dietary Fiber: 8g
- Sugars: 10g
- Total Fat: 15g
- Saturated Fat: 3g
- Sodium: 200mg

Serves:

- **2 servings**

Cooking Time:

- **Total: 20 minutes**

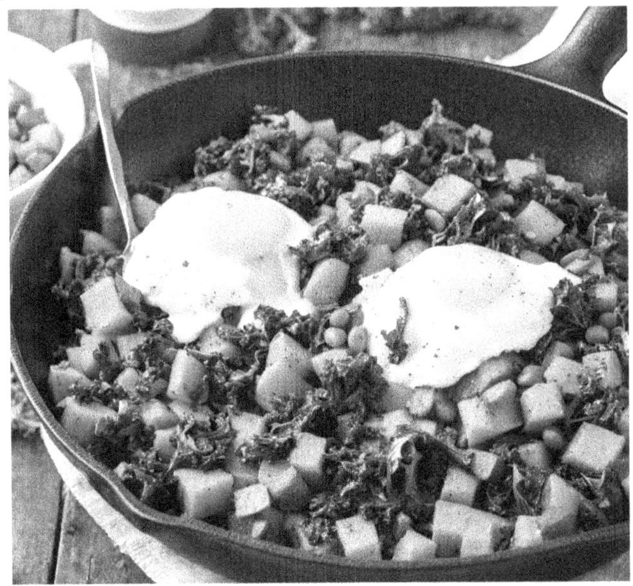

4. Millet Breakfast Bowl

Ingredients:

- 1 cup of millet
- 2 cups of water
- 1/2 cup of unsweetened almond milk
- 1 tablespoon of honey or maple syrup
- 1/4 cup of chopped nuts (e.g., almonds or walnuts)
- 1/4 cup of dried cranberries
- 1 teaspoon of ground cinnamon
- Fresh fruit (e.g., sliced banana, berries) for topping

Instructions:

1. Rinse the millet under cold water.
2. In a medium saucepan, bring the water to a boil.
3. Add the millet to the boiling water, reduce the heat to low, and simmer for about 20 minutes or until the millet is tender and the water is absorbed.
4. Stir in the almond milk, honey or maple syrup, chopped nuts, dried cranberries, and ground cinnamon.
5. Cook for an additional 2-3 minutes until heated through.
6. Serve topped with fresh fruit.

Nutrition Info (Per Serving):

- Calories: 280
- Protein: 7g
- Carbohydrates: 45g
- Dietary Fiber: 5g
- Sugars: 15g
- Total Fat: 9g
- Saturated Fat: 1g
- Sodium: 10mg

Serves:

- 4 servings

Cooking Time:

- **Total: 30 minutes**

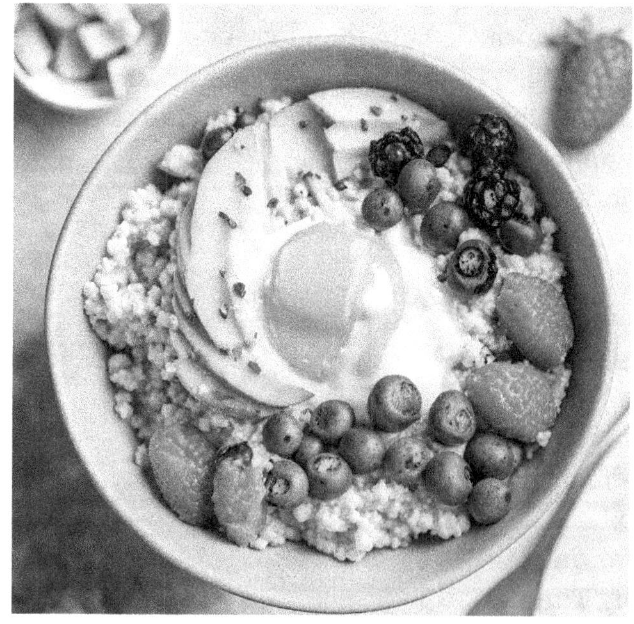

5. Soy Yogurt with Mixed Berries

Ingredients:

- 2 cups of plain soy yogurt
- 1 cup of mixed berries (e.g., strawberries, blueberries, raspberries)
- 1 tablespoon of honey or maple syrup
- 1/4 cup of granola (optional)
- 1 tablespoon of chia seeds (optional)

Instructions:

1. Divide the soy yogurt into two bowls.
2. Top each bowl with mixed berries.
3. Drizzle with honey or maple syrup.
4. Sprinkle with granola and chia seeds if using.
5. Serve immediately.

Nutrition Info (Per Serving):

- Calories: 200
- Protein: 6g
- Carbohydrates: 30g
- Dietary Fiber: 5g
- Sugars: 15g
- Total Fat: 6g
- Saturated Fat: 1g
- Sodium: 50mg

Serves:

- **2 servings**

Cooking Time:

- **Total: 5 minutes**

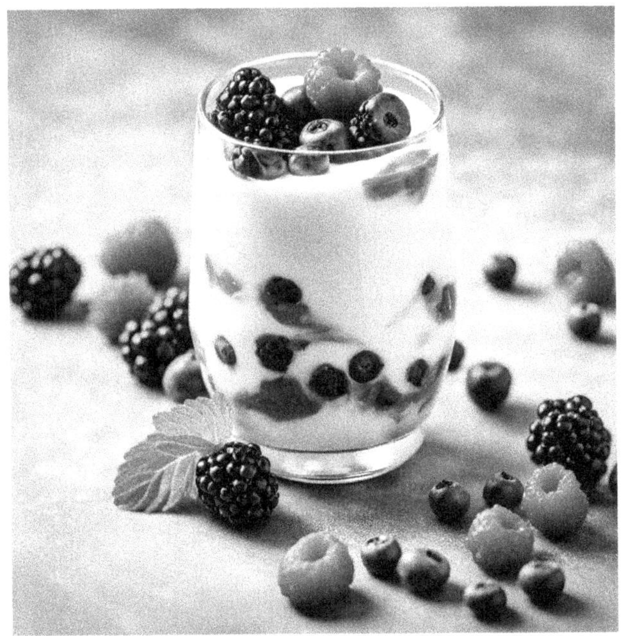

6. Stewed Prunes

Ingredients:

- 2 cups of pitted prunes
- 2 cups of water
- 1 teaspoon of ground cinnamon
- 1 teaspoon of vanilla extract

Instructions:

1. In a medium saucepan, combine the prunes, water, ground cinnamon, and vanilla extract.
2. Bring to a boil over medium-high heat.
3. Reduce the heat to low and simmer for about 20 minutes, or until the prunes are tender and the liquid has thickened.
4. Let cool slightly before serving.

Nutrition Info (Per Serving):

- Calories: 180
- Protein: 1g
- Carbohydrates: 48g
- Dietary Fiber: 6g
- Sugars: 40g
- Total Fat: 0g
- Saturated Fat: 0g
- Sodium: 5mg

Serves:

- **4 servings**

Cooking Time:

- **Total: 25 minutes**

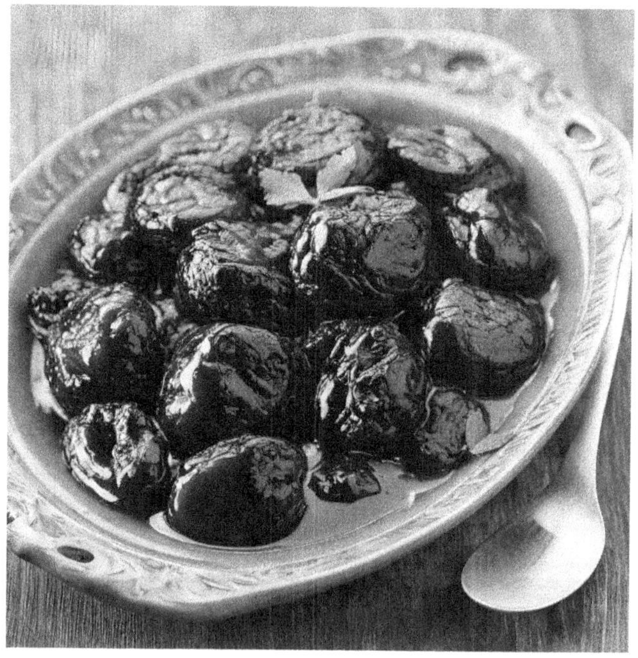

7. Zucchini Bread

Ingredients:

- 1 1/2 cups of whole wheat flour
- 1 teaspoon of baking soda
- 1 teaspoon of ground cinnamon
- 1/2 teaspoon of ground nutmeg
- 1/4 teaspoon of salt
- 2 large eggs
- 1/2 cup of unsweetened applesauce
- 1/4 cup of honey or maple syrup
- 1/4 cup of olive oil
- 1 teaspoon of vanilla extract
- 1 1/2 cups of grated zucchini

Instructions:

1. Preheat the oven to 350°F (175°C). Grease a 9x5-inch loaf pan.
2. In a large bowl, whisk together the flour, baking soda, ground cinnamon, ground nutmeg, and salt.
3. In another bowl, beat the eggs and mix in the applesauce, honey or maple syrup, olive oil, and vanilla extract.
4. Stir the wet ingredients into the dry ingredients until just combined.
5. Fold in the grated zucchini.
6. Pour the batter into the prepared loaf pan and smooth the top.
7. Bake for 50-60 minutes, or until a toothpick inserted into the center comes out clean.
8. Let cool in the pan for 10 minutes, then transfer to a wire rack to cool completely.

Nutrition Info (Per Serving):

- Calories: 200
- Protein: 4g
- Carbohydrates: 30g
- Dietary Fiber: 4g
- Sugars: 10g
- Total Fat: 8g
- Saturated Fat: 1g
- Sodium: 150mg

Serves:

- **10 servings**

Cooking Time:

- **Total: 70 minutes**

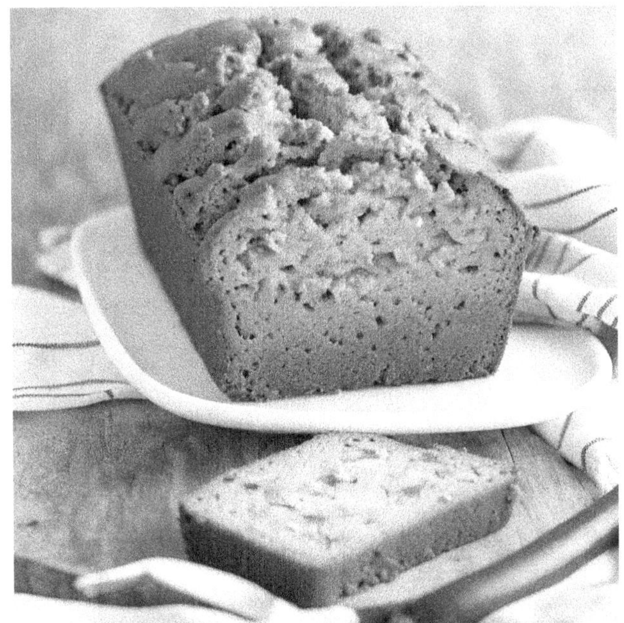

8. Sweet Corn Porridge

Ingredients:

- 1 cup of cornmeal
- 4 cups of water
- 1/2 cup of unsweetened almond milk
- 1 tablespoon of honey or maple syrup
- 1 teaspoon of vanilla extract
- Fresh fruit (e.g., sliced banana, berries) for topping

Instructions:

1. In a medium saucepan, bring the water to a boil.
2. Gradually whisk in the cornmeal, reducing the heat to low.
3. Cook, stirring frequently, for about 20 minutes or until the mixture thickens and the cornmeal is tender.
4. Stir in the almond milk, honey or maple syrup, and vanilla extract.
5. Cook for an additional 2-3 minutes until heated through.
6. Serve topped with fresh fruit.

Nutrition Info (Per Serving):

- Calories: 180
- Protein: 3g
- Carbohydrates: 35g
- Dietary Fiber: 3g
- Sugars: 10g
- Total Fat: 3g
- Saturated Fat: 0g
- Sodium: 10mg

Serves:

- **4 servings**

Cooking Time:

- **Total: 25 minutes**

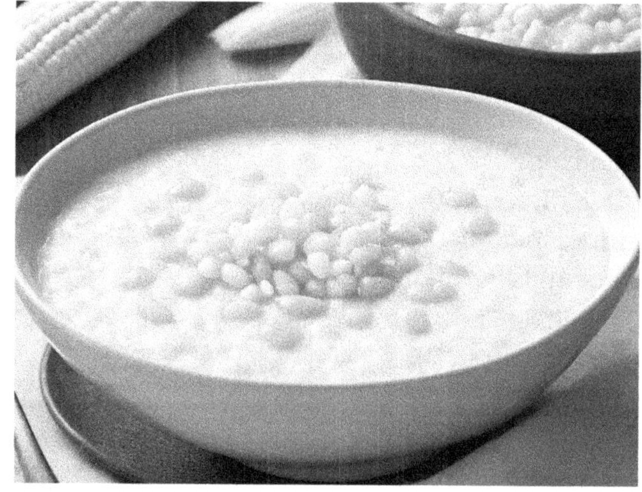

9. Cucumber and Carrot Juice

Ingredients:

- 2 medium cucumbers
- 4 large carrots
- 1 apple (optional for sweetness)
- 1 inch of fresh ginger (optional for flavor)
- 1 cup of water

Instructions:

1. Wash the cucumbers, carrots, and apple thoroughly.
2. Peel the carrots and cut all the ingredients into pieces that will fit your juicer.
3. If using, peel and grate the ginger.
4. Place the cucumbers, carrots, apple, and ginger into the juicer.
5. Add the cup of water to help with the juicing process.
6. Serve the juice immediately over ice, if desired.

Nutrition Info (Per Serving):

- Calories: 80
- Protein: 1g
- Carbohydrates: 20g
- Dietary Fiber: 5g
- Sugars: 15g
- Total Fat: 0g
- Saturated Fat: 0g
- Sodium: 50mg

Serves:

- 2 servings

Cooking Time:

- **Total: 10 minutes**

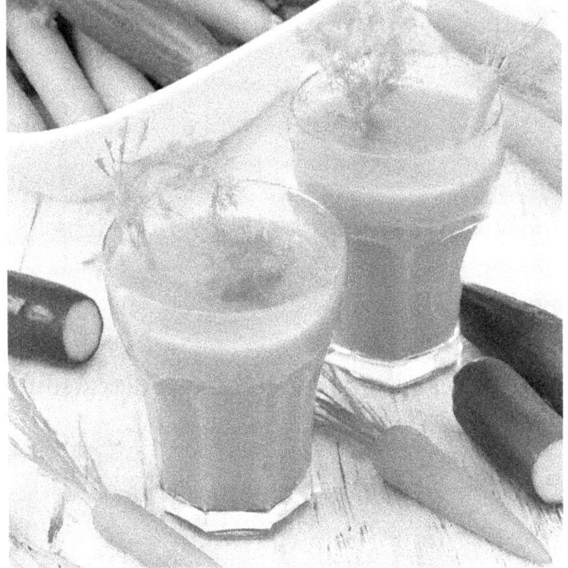

10. Bircher Muesli

Ingredients:

- 1 cup of rolled oats
- 1 cup of unsweetened almond milk
- 1/2 cup of plain yogurt (dairy or soy)
- 1 apple, grated
- 1/4 cup of raisins
- 1 tablespoon of chia seeds
- 1 tablespoon of honey or maple syrup
- 1/2 teaspoon of ground cinnamon
- Fresh berries for topping

Instructions:

1. In a large bowl, combine the rolled oats, almond milk, yogurt, grated apple, raisins, chia seeds, honey or maple syrup, and ground cinnamon.
2. Mix well until all ingredients are evenly distributed.
3. Cover the bowl and refrigerate overnight.
4. In the morning, stir the muesli and add a bit more milk if it's too thick.
5. Serve topped with fresh berries.

Nutrition Info (Per Serving):

- Calories: 220
- Protein: 6g
- Carbohydrates: 45g
- Dietary Fiber: 7g
- Sugars: 15g
- Total Fat: 5g
- Saturated Fat: 1g
- Sodium: 40mg

Serves:

- **4 servings**

Cooking Time:

- **Total: 10 minutes (plus overnight refrigeration)**

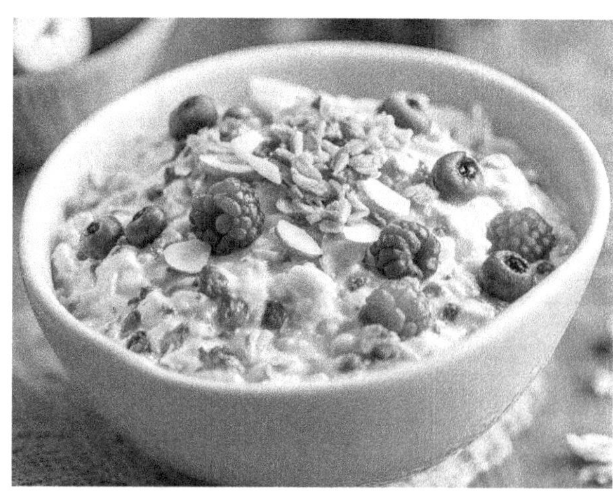

12. Smooth Cottage Cheese with Blueberries

Ingredients:

- 2 cups of cottage cheese (low-fat)
- 1 cup of fresh blueberries
- 1 tablespoon of honey or maple syrup
- 1/2 teaspoon of vanilla extract
- Fresh mint leaves for garnish (optional)

Instructions:

1. In a blender, combine the cottage cheese, honey or maple syrup, and vanilla extract.
2. Blend until smooth and creamy.
3. Divide the cottage cheese mixture into bowls.
4. Top with fresh blueberries and garnish with mint leaves if desired.
5. Serve immediately.

Nutrition Info (Per Serving):

- Calories: 150
- Protein: 14g
- Carbohydrates: 18g
- Dietary Fiber: 2g
- Sugars: 12g
- Total Fat: 3g
- Saturated Fat: 1g
- Sodium: 400mg

Serves:

- 2 servings

Cooking Time:

- **Total: 5 minutes**

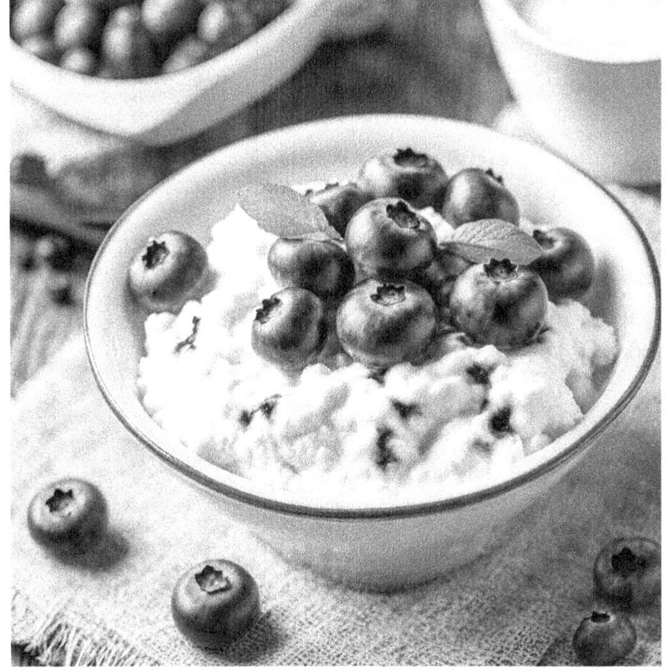

13. Pear and Ginger Muffins

Ingredients:

- 1 1/2 cups of whole wheat flour
- 1 teaspoon of baking powder
- 1/2 teaspoon of baking soda
- 1 teaspoon of ground ginger
- 1/4 teaspoon of ground cinnamon
- 2 large eggs
- 1/2 cup of unsweetened applesauce
- 1/4 cup of honey or maple syrup
- 1/4 cup of olive oil
- 1 teaspoon of vanilla extract
- 1 cup of finely chopped pears (peeled)

Instructions:

1. Preheat the oven to 350°F (175°C). Line a muffin tin with paper liners.
2. In a large bowl, whisk together the flour, baking powder, baking soda, ground ginger, and ground cinnamon.
3. In another bowl, beat the eggs and mix in the applesauce, honey or maple syrup, olive oil, and vanilla extract.
4. Stir the wet ingredients into the dry ingredients until just combined.
5. Fold in the chopped pears.
6. Divide the batter evenly among the muffin cups.
7. Bake for 18-20 minutes, or until a toothpick inserted into the center comes out clean.
8. Let cool in the tin for 5 minutes, then transfer to a wire rack to cool completely.

Nutrition Info (Per Serving):

- Calories: 160
- Protein: 4g
- Carbohydrates: 28g
- Dietary Fiber: 3g
- Sugars: 12g
- Total Fat: 5g
- Saturated Fat: 1g
- Sodium: 150mg

Serves:

- **12 muffins**

Cooking Time:

- **Total: 30 minutes**

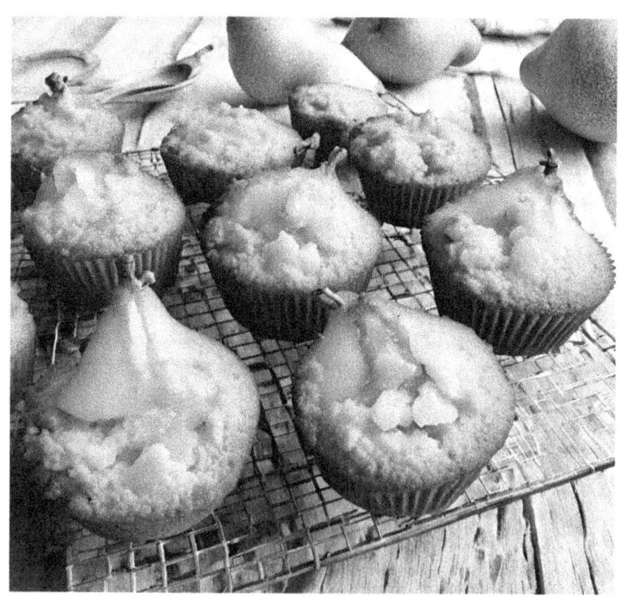

14. Barley Soup

Ingredients:

- 1 cup of pearl barley
- 6 cups of low-sodium vegetable broth
- 2 medium carrots, diced
- 2 celery stalks, diced
- 1 medium potato, diced
- 1 cup of chopped kale (if tolerated, cooked)
- 1 tablespoon of olive oil
- 1 teaspoon of dried thyme
- 1 bay leaf

Instructions:

1. Rinse the pearl barley under cold water.
2. In a large pot, heat the olive oil over medium heat.
3. Add the diced carrots, celery, and potato. Cook for 5-7 minutes until vegetables are slightly softened.
4. Add the vegetable broth, barley, thyme, and bay leaf. Bring to a boil.
5. Reduce heat to low and simmer for 45-50 minutes, or until the barley is tender.
6. Remove the bay leaf and stir in the chopped kale (if tolerated).
7. Cook for an additional 5 minutes.
8. Serve warm.

Nutrition Info (Per Serving):

- Calories: 200
- Protein: 5g
- Carbohydrates: 40g
- Dietary Fiber: 8g
- Sugars: 4g
- Total Fat: 4g
- Saturated Fat: 0.5g
- Sodium: 150mg

Serves:

- **6 servings**

Cooking Time:

- **Total: 1 hour**

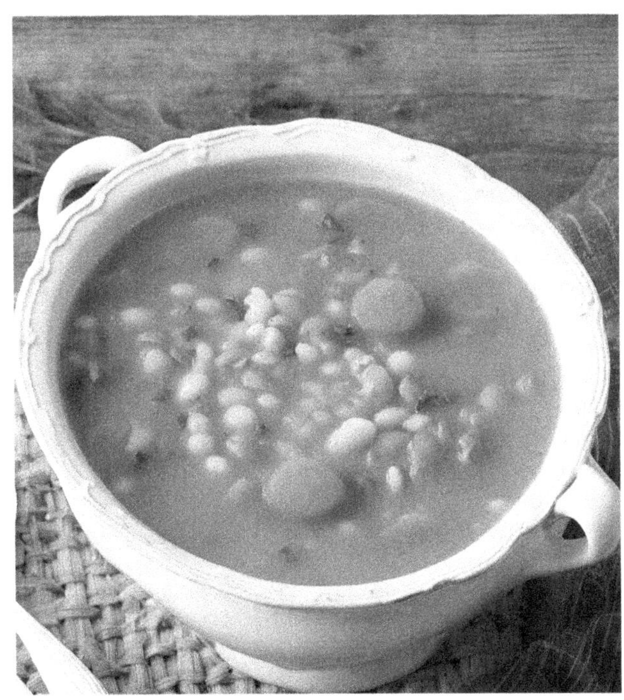

15. Buckwheat Crepes

Ingredients:

- 1 cup of buckwheat flour
- 1 1/4 cups of unsweetened almond milk
- 2 large eggs
- 2 tablespoons of olive oil
- 1 teaspoon of honey or maple syrup
- 1/2 teaspoon of ground cinnamon

Instructions:

1. In a large bowl, whisk together the buckwheat flour, almond milk, eggs, olive oil, honey or maple syrup, and ground cinnamon until smooth.
2. Heat a non-stick skillet over medium heat and lightly grease with olive oil.
3. Pour 1/4 cup of batter into the skillet and tilt the pan to spread the batter evenly.
4. Cook for 1-2 minutes on each side, or until the crepe is lightly golden.
5. Repeat with the remaining batter.
6. Serve warm, with desired toppings such as fresh fruit or yogurt.

Nutrition Info (Per Serving):

- Calories: 150
- Protein: 6g
- Carbohydrates: 20g
- Dietary Fiber: 3g
- Sugars: 3g
- Total Fat: 5g
- Saturated Fat: 1g
- Sodium: 60mg

Serves:

- **6 crepes**

Cooking Time: Total: 20 minutes

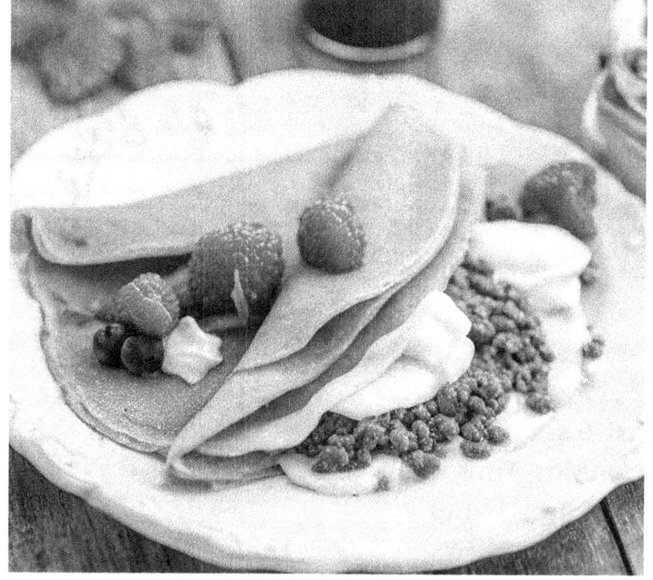

16. Multigrain Waffles

Ingredients:

- 1 cup of whole wheat flour
- 1/2 cup of oat flour
- 1/2 cup of cornmeal
- 2 tablespoons of flaxseed meal
- 1 1/2 cups of unsweetened almond milk
- 2 large eggs
- 2 tablespoons of olive oil
- 1 tablespoon of honey or maple syrup
- 1 teaspoon of baking powder
- 1/2 teaspoon of ground cinnamon

Instructions:

1. In a large bowl, combine the whole wheat flour, oat flour, cornmeal, flaxseed meal, baking powder, and ground cinnamon.
2. In another bowl, whisk together the almond milk, eggs, olive oil, and honey or maple syrup.
3. Stir the wet ingredients into the dry ingredients until just combined.
4. Preheat a waffle iron and lightly grease with olive oil.
5. Pour the batter into the preheated waffle iron and cook according to the manufacturer's instructions until golden brown and crisp.
6. Serve with fresh fruit or a drizzle of honey or maple syrup.

Nutrition Info (Per Serving):

- Calories: 180
- Protein: 6g
- Carbohydrates: 30g
- Dietary Fiber: 5g
- Sugars: 5g
- Total Fat: 5g
- Saturated Fat: 1g
- Sodium: 100mg

Serves:

- **6 waffles**

Cooking Time:

- **Total: 25 minutes**

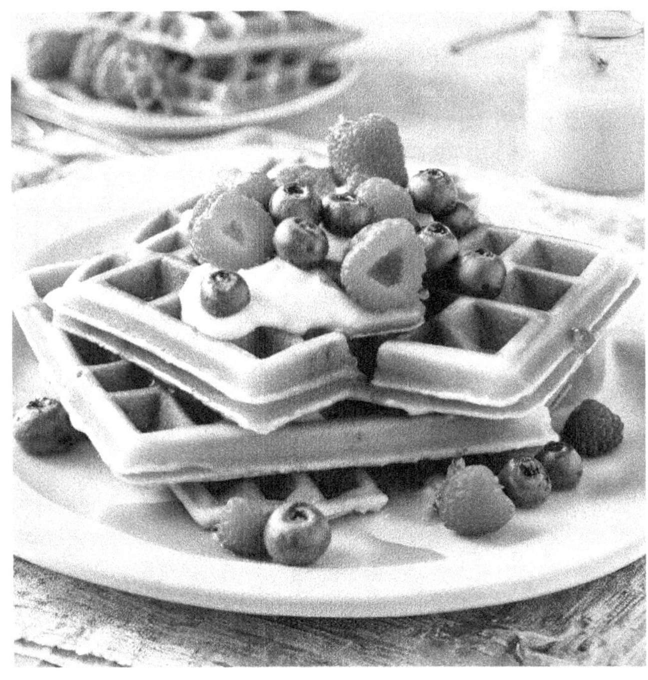

17. Rice Cakes with Avocado

Ingredients:

- 6 plain rice cakes
- 2 ripe avocados
- 1 tablespoon of lemon juice (if tolerated)
- 1 teaspoon of olive oil
- 1/4 teaspoon of ground cumin
- Fresh herbs (e.g., parsley, cilantro) for garnish

Instructions:

1. In a bowl, mash the avocados with lemon juice (if tolerated), olive oil, and ground cumin until smooth.
2. Spread the avocado mixture evenly over the rice cakes.
3. Garnish with fresh herbs.
4. Serve immediately.

Nutrition Info (Per Serving):

- Calories: 150
- Protein: 2g
- Carbohydrates: 20g
- Dietary Fiber: 5g
- Sugars: 0g
- Total Fat: 8g
- Saturated Fat: 1g
- Sodium: 10mg

Serves:

- **6 servings**

Cooking Time:

- **Total: 10 minutes**

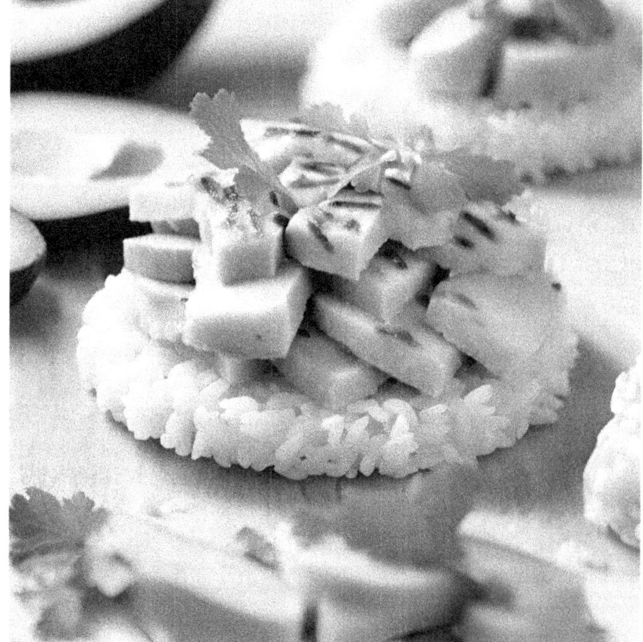

18. Quinoa Porridge

Ingredients:

- 1 cup of quinoa
- 2 cups of unsweetened almond milk
- 1 tablespoon of honey or maple syrup
- 1 teaspoon of vanilla extract
- 1/2 teaspoon of ground cinnamon
- Fresh berries for topping

Instructions:

1. Rinse the quinoa under cold water.
2. In a medium saucepan, combine the quinoa and almond milk. Bring to a boil.
3. Reduce heat to low and simmer for about 15 minutes, or until the quinoa is tender and the liquid is absorbed.
4. Stir in the honey or maple syrup, vanilla extract, and ground cinnamon.
5. Serve topped with fresh berries.

Nutrition Info (Per Serving):

- Calories: 200
- Protein: 6g
- Carbohydrates: 35g
- Dietary Fiber: 5g
- Sugars: 10g
- Total Fat: 4g
- Saturated Fat: 0g
- Sodium: 40mg

Serves:

- **4 servings**

Cooking Time:

- **Total: 20 minutes**

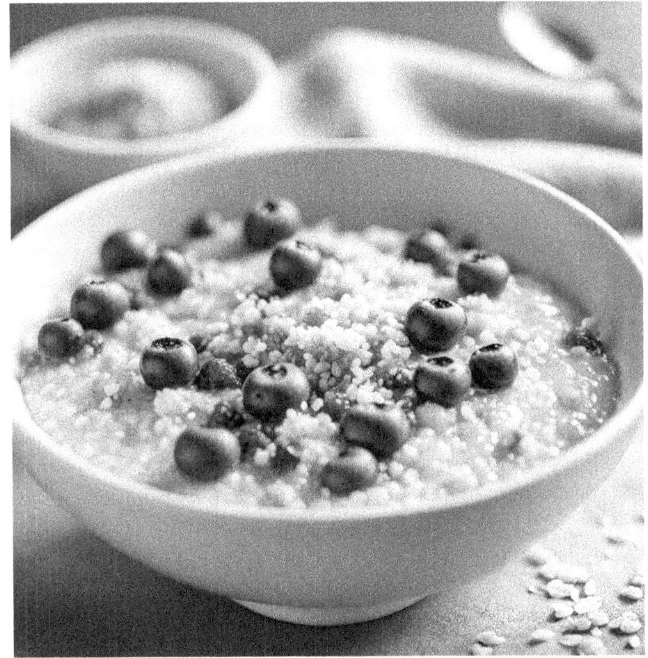

19. Almond Milk Smoothie

Ingredients:

- 1 cup of unsweetened almond milk
- 1 banana, frozen
- 1/2 cup of frozen berries
- 1 tablespoon of chia seeds
- 1 teaspoon of honey or maple syrup
- 1/2 teaspoon of vanilla extract

Instructions:

1. Combine all ingredients in a blender.
2. Blend until smooth and creamy.
3. Pour into a glass and serve immediately.

Nutrition Info (Per Serving):

- Calories: 150
- Protein: 3g
- Carbohydrates: 30g
- Dietary Fiber: 6g
- Sugars: 15g
- Total Fat: 4g
- Saturated Fat: 0g
- Sodium: 100mg

Serves:

- **1 serving**

Cooking Time:

- **Total: 5 minutes**

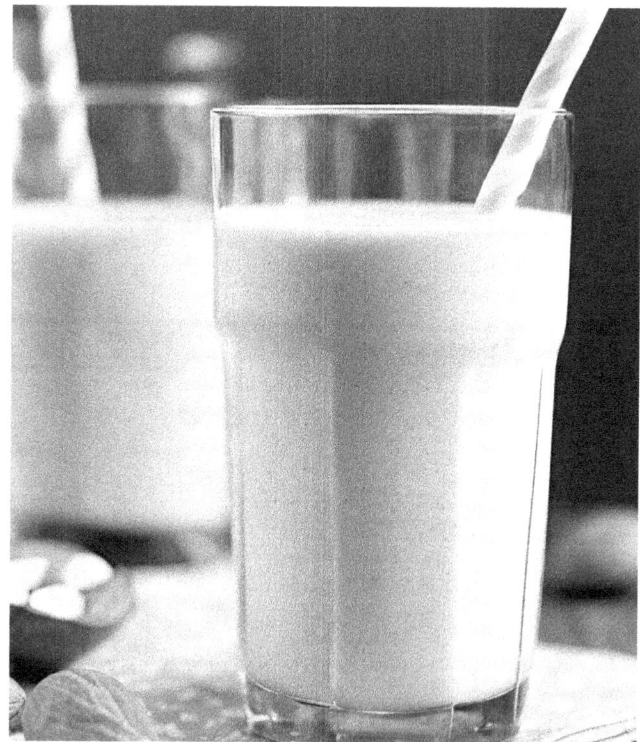

20. Vegetable Omelette

Ingredients:

- 3 large eggs
- 1/4 cup of unsweetened almond milk
- 1/2 cup of diced zucchini
- 1/2 cup of diced mushrooms
- 1/4 cup of fresh spinach (chopped)
- 1 tablespoon of olive oil
- 1/4 cup of grated low-fat cheese (optional)
- Fresh herbs (e.g., parsley, chives) for garnish

Instructions:

1. In a bowl, whisk together the eggs and almond milk until well combined.
2. Heat the olive oil in a non-stick skillet over medium heat.
3. Add the diced zucchini and mushrooms to the skillet and sauté for 4-5 minutes until tender.
4. Pour the egg mixture over the vegetables and cook until the edges start to set.
5. Sprinkle with fresh spinach and grated cheese (if using).
6. Cover and cook for an additional 3-4 minutes, until the omelette is fully set.
7. Garnish with fresh herbs before serving.

Nutrition Info (Per Serving):

- Calories: 220
- Protein: 14g
- Carbohydrates: 5g
- Dietary Fiber: 1g
- Sugars: 2g
- Total Fat: 16g
- Saturated Fat: 4g
- Sodium: 150mg

Serves:

- **2 servings**

Cooking Time:

- **Total: 15 minutes**

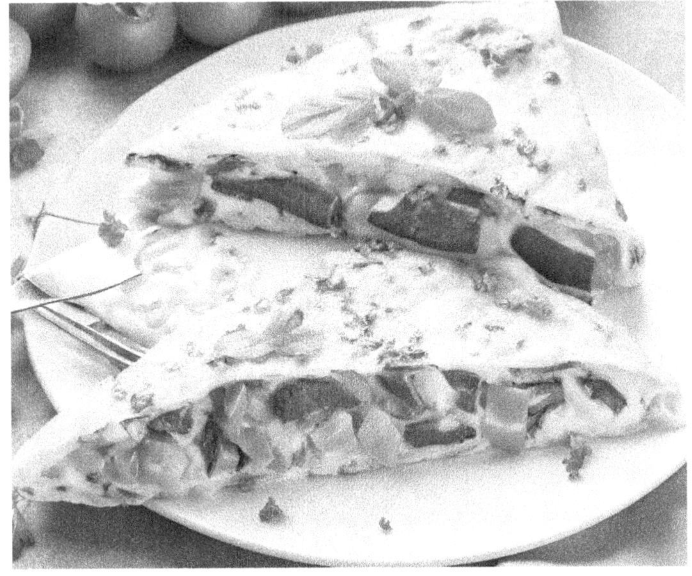

21. Steamed Rice with Poached Chicken

Ingredients:

- 1 cup of jasmine rice
- 2 cups of water
- 2 boneless, skinless chicken breasts
- 4 cups of low-sodium chicken broth
- 1 teaspoon of dried thyme
- 1 teaspoon of dried oregano
- Fresh parsley for garnish

Instructions:

1. Rinse the jasmine rice under cold water.
2. In a medium saucepan, bring the water to a boil.
3. Add the rice, reduce heat to low, cover, and simmer for 15-20 minutes, until the rice is tender and the water is absorbed.
4. In another pot, bring the chicken broth to a gentle simmer.
5. Add the chicken breasts, thyme, and oregano to the broth.
6. Poach the chicken for 15-20 minutes, until fully cooked.
7. Remove the chicken from the broth and let rest for a few minutes before slicing.
8. Serve the steamed rice with the poached chicken, garnished with fresh parsley.

Nutrition Info (Per Serving):

- Calories: 350
- Protein: 28g
- Carbohydrates: 40g
- Dietary Fiber: 1g
- Sugars: 0g
- Total Fat: 6g
- Saturated Fat: 1g
- Sodium: 200mg

Serves:

- **4 servings**

Cooking Time:

- **Total: 30 minutes**

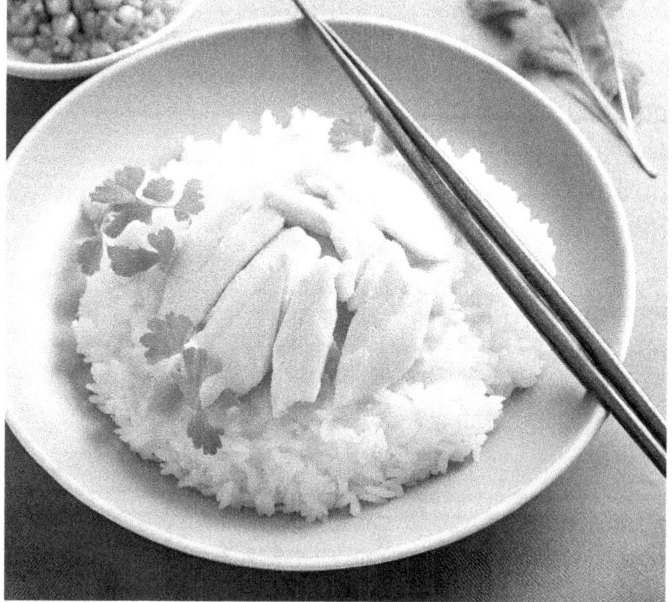

22. Sweet Potato Hash

Ingredients:

- 2 medium sweet potatoes, peeled and diced
- 1 tablespoon of olive oil
- 1/2 cup of diced mushrooms
- 1/2 cup of diced zucchini
- 1/4 teaspoon of ground cumin
- Fresh parsley for garnish

Instructions:

1. Heat the olive oil in a large skillet over medium heat.
2. Add the diced sweet potatoes to the skillet and cook for 10-12 minutes, stirring occasionally, until tender and slightly crispy.
3. Add the mushrooms and zucchini to the skillet and cook for an additional 5 minutes.
4. Sprinkle with ground cumin and stir to combine.
5. Garnish with fresh parsley before serving.

Nutrition Info (Per Serving):

- Calories: 180
- Protein: 2g
- Carbohydrates: 32g
- Dietary Fiber: 5g
- Sugars: 8g
- Total Fat: 6g
- Saturated Fat: 1g
- Sodium: 50mg

Serves:

- **4 servings**

Cooking Time:

- **Total: 20 minutes**

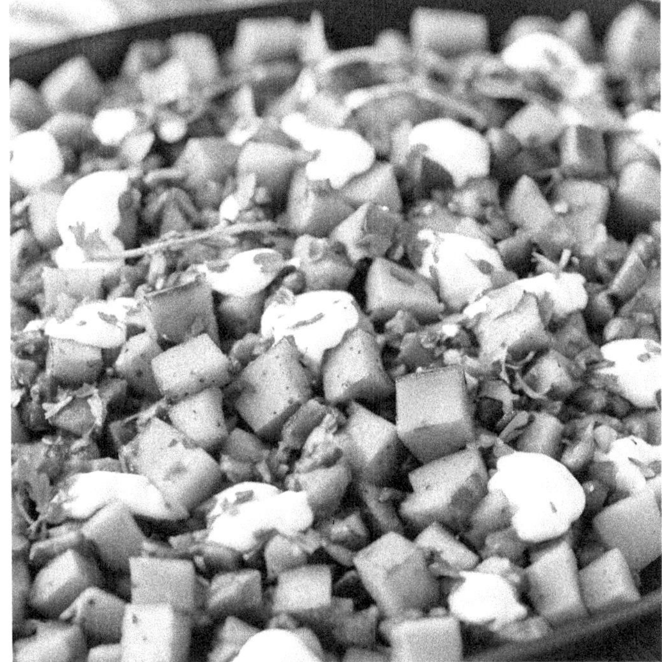

23. Pumpkin Pancakes

Ingredients:

- 1 cup of whole wheat flour
- 1 tablespoon of baking powder
- 1 teaspoon of ground cinnamon
- 1/2 teaspoon of ground nutmeg
- 1/4 teaspoon of ground ginger
- 1/2 cup of canned pumpkin puree
- 1 cup of unsweetened almond milk
- 1 large egg
- 2 tablespoons of honey or maple syrup
- 1 tablespoon of olive oil

Instructions:

1. In a large bowl, whisk together the flour, baking powder, ground cinnamon, ground nutmeg, and ground ginger.
2. In another bowl, mix the pumpkin puree, almond milk, egg, honey or maple syrup, and olive oil until smooth.
3. Stir the wet ingredients into the dry ingredients until just combined.
4. Heat a non-stick skillet or griddle over medium heat and lightly grease with olive oil.
5. Pour 1/4 cup of batter onto the skillet and cook for 2-3 minutes on each side, until golden brown.
6. Serve warm, with a drizzle of honey or maple syrup if desired.

Nutrition Info (Per Serving):

- Calories: 120
- Protein: 4g
- Carbohydrates: 20g
- Dietary Fiber: 3g
- Sugars: 7g
- Total Fat: 4g
- Saturated Fat: 1g
- Sodium: 150mg

Serves:

- **8 pancakes**

Cooking Time:

- **Total: 20 minutes**

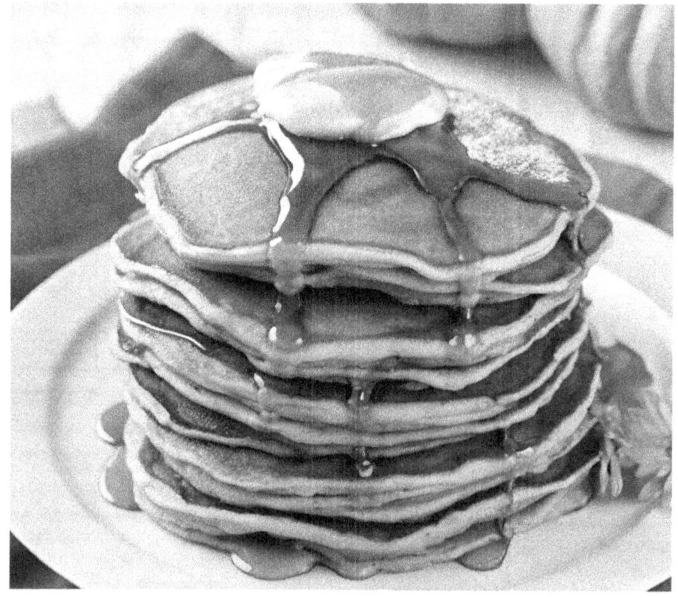

24. Apple Cinnamon Rice

Ingredients:

- 1 cup of basmati rice
- 2 cups of water
- 2 apples, peeled and diced
- 1/2 teaspoon of ground cinnamon
- 1/4 cup of raisins
- 1 tablespoon of honey or maple syrup

Instructions:

1. Rinse the basmati rice under cold water.
2. In a medium saucepan, bring the water to a boil.
3. Add the rice, reduce heat to low, cover, and simmer for 15 minutes.
4. Add the diced apples, ground cinnamon, raisins, and honey or maple syrup to the rice.
5. Stir to combine and cook for an additional 5 minutes, until the apples are tender.
6. Serve warm.

Nutrition Info (Per Serving):

- Calories: 180
- Protein: 2g
- Carbohydrates: 40g
- Dietary Fiber: 3g
- Sugars: 15g
- Total Fat: 1g
- Saturated Fat: 0g
- Sodium: 10mg

Serves:

- **4 servings**

Cooking Time:

- **Total: 25 minutes**

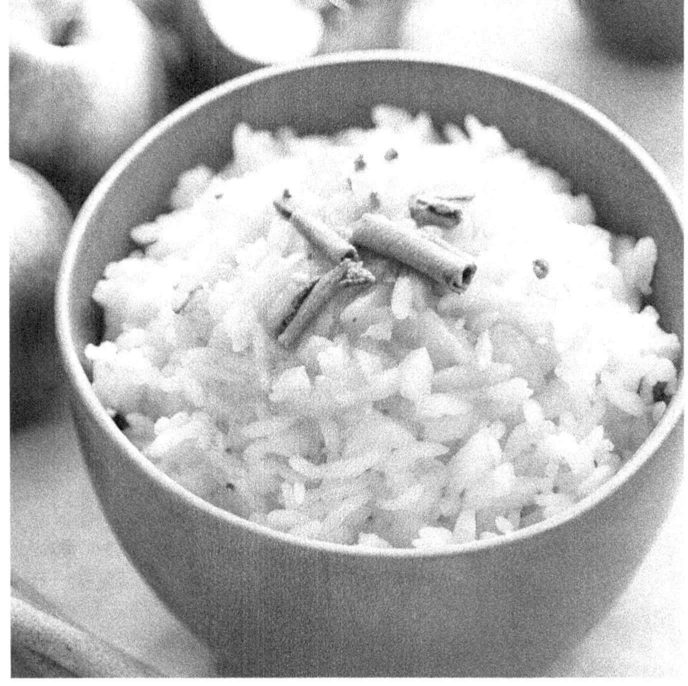

25. Banana Yogurt Smoothie

Ingredients:

- 1 cup of plain yogurt (dairy or soy)
- 1 ripe banana
- 1/2 cup of unsweetened almond milk
- 1 tablespoon of honey or maple syrup
- 1/2 teaspoon of vanilla extract

Instructions:

1. Combine all ingredients in a blender.
2. Blend until smooth and creamy.
3. Pour into a glass and serve immediately.

Nutrition Info (Per Serving):

- Calories: 200
- Protein: 6g
- Carbohydrates: 40g
- Dietary Fiber: 3g
- Sugars: 25g
- Total Fat: 4g
- Saturated Fat: 1g
- Sodium: 100mg

Serves:

- **2 servings**

Cooking Time:

- **Total: 5 minutes**

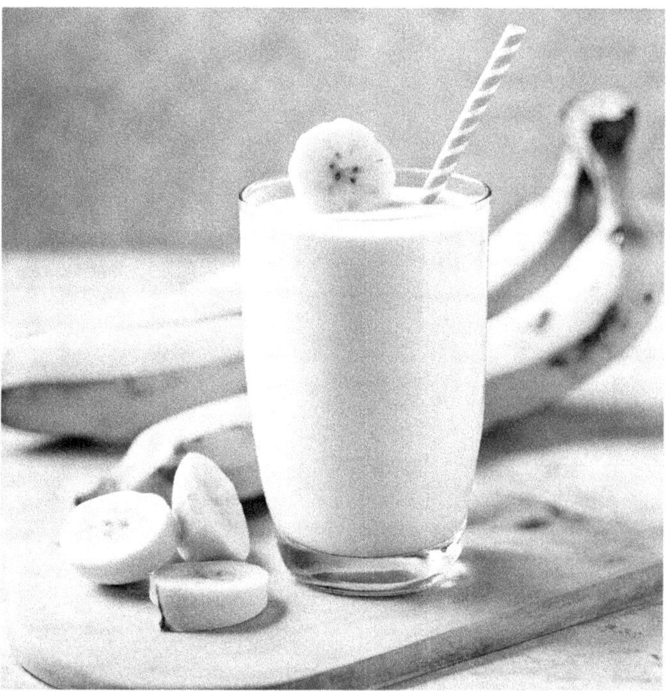

26. Oatmeal Porridge

Ingredients:
- 1 cup of rolled oats
- 2 cups of unsweetened almond milk
- 1 tablespoon of honey or maple syrup
- 1/2 teaspoon of ground cinnamon
- 1/4 cup of chopped nuts (e.g., almonds or walnuts)
- Fresh berries for topping

Instructions:
1. In a medium saucepan, bring the almond milk to a gentle boil.
2. Stir in the rolled oats and reduce heat to low.
3. Cook, stirring occasionally, for about 5-7 minutes until the oats are tender and the porridge is creamy.
4. Stir in the honey or maple syrup and ground cinnamon.
5. Serve topped with chopped nuts and fresh berries.

Nutrition Info (Per Serving):
- Calories: 250
- Protein: 6g
- Carbohydrates: 40g
- Dietary Fiber: 6g
- Sugars: 10g
- Total Fat: 8g
- Saturated Fat: 1g
- Sodium: 100mg

Serves:
- **2 servings**

Cooking Time:
- **Total: 10 minutes**

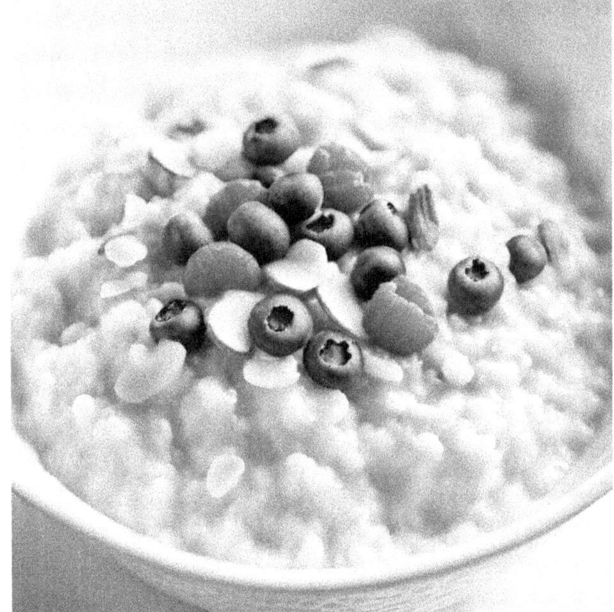

Fish & Seafood Recipes

1. Steamed Salmon with Dill

Ingredients:

- 4 salmon fillets (about 6 ounces each)
- 1 tablespoon of olive oil
- 1/4 cup of fresh dill, chopped
- 1/2 cup of low-sodium vegetable broth
- 1 lemon, thinly sliced (if tolerated)
- Fresh parsley for garnish

Instructions:

1. Brush the salmon fillets with olive oil and sprinkle with fresh dill.
2. Place the salmon fillets in a steamer basket over simmering water or vegetable broth.
3. Add the lemon slices (if tolerated) on top of the salmon.
4. Cover and steam for about 8-10 minutes, or until the salmon is cooked through and flakes easily with a fork.
5. Garnish with fresh parsley before serving.

Nutrition Info (Per Serving):

- Calories: 290
- Protein: 25g
- Carbohydrates: 2g
- Dietary Fiber: 0g
- Sugars: 0g
- Total Fat: 20g
- Saturated Fat: 3g
- Sodium: 70mg

Serves:

- **4 servings**

Cooking Time:

- **Total: 15 minutes**

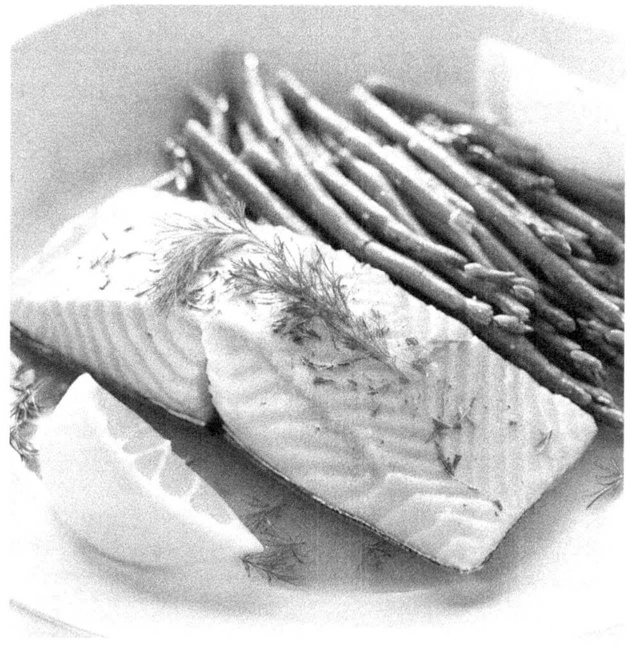

2. Baked Tilapia with Herbs

Ingredients:

- 4 tilapia fillets (about 6 ounces each)
- 2 tablespoons of olive oil
- 1 teaspoon of dried thyme
- 1 teaspoon of dried oregano
- 1 teaspoon of dried basil
- 1/2 cup of low-sodium vegetable broth
- Fresh parsley for garnish

Instructions:

1. Preheat the oven to 375°F (190°C).
2. Brush the tilapia fillets with olive oil.
3. Sprinkle the fillets with dried thyme, oregano, and basil.
4. Place the fillets in a baking dish and pour the vegetable broth around them.
5. Bake for 15-20 minutes, or until the fish is opaque and flakes easily with a fork.
6. Garnish with fresh parsley before serving.

Nutrition Info (Per Serving):

- Calories: 200
- Protein: 30g
- Carbohydrates: 1g
- Dietary Fiber: 0g
- Sugars: 0g
- Total Fat: 8g
- Saturated Fat: 1g
- Sodium: 100mg

Serves:

- **4 servings**

Cooking Time:

- **Total: 25 minutes**

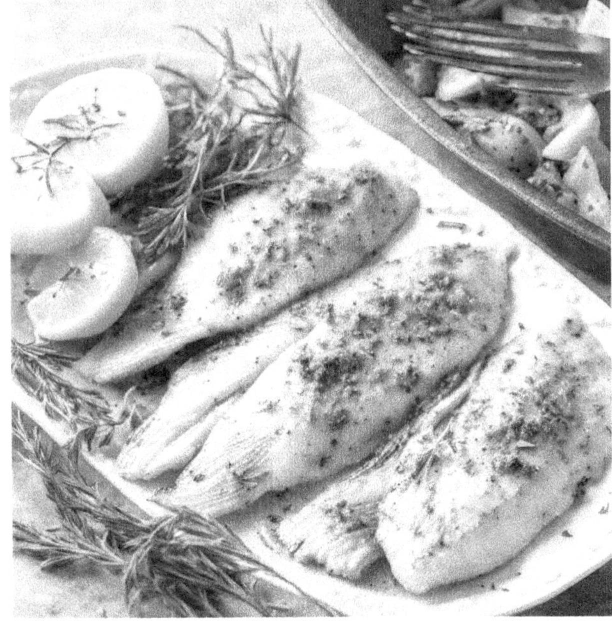

3. Poached Cod

Ingredients:
- 4 cod fillets (about 6 ounces each)
- 4 cups of low-sodium vegetable broth
- 1 tablespoon of olive oil
- 1 teaspoon of dried thyme
- 1 teaspoon of dried parsley
- 1 bay leaf

Instructions:
1. In a large pot, bring the vegetable broth to a simmer.
2. Add the olive oil, dried thyme, dried parsley, and bay leaf to the broth.
3. Gently place the cod fillets into the simmering broth.
4. Poach the cod for 8-10 minutes, or until the fish is opaque and flakes easily with a fork.
5. Remove the bay leaf and serve the cod with a bit of the poaching liquid.

Nutrition Info (Per Serving):
- Calories: 160
- Protein: 32g
- Carbohydrates: 1g
- Dietary Fiber: 0g
- Sugars: 0g
- Total Fat: 3g
- Saturated Fat: 0.5g
- Sodium: 100mg

Serves:
- **4 servings**

Cooking Time:
- **Total: 15 minutes**

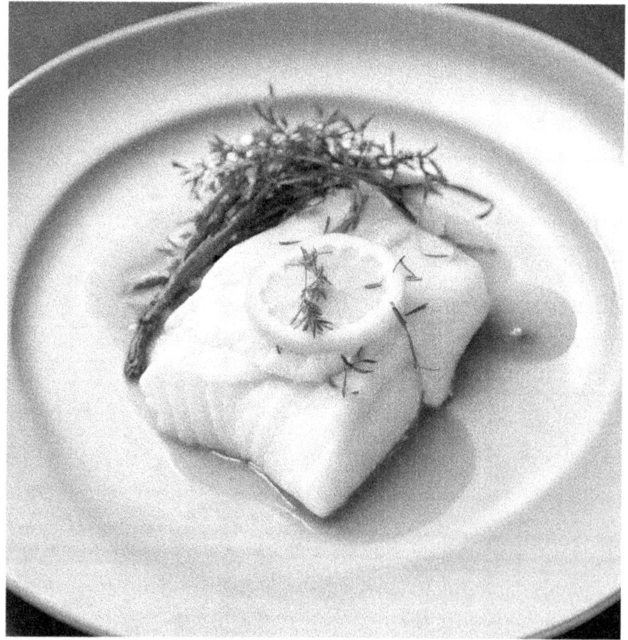

4. Shrimp and Rice Soup

Ingredients:

- 1 cup of jasmine rice
- 1 pound of shrimp, peeled and deveined
- 6 cups of low-sodium chicken or vegetable broth
- 2 medium carrots, diced
- 2 celery stalks, diced
- 1 tablespoon of olive oil
- 1 teaspoon of dried thyme
- Fresh parsley for garnish

Instructions:

1. In a large pot, heat the olive oil over medium heat.
2. Add the diced carrots and celery, and sauté for 5 minutes until slightly softened.
3. Add the broth and bring to a boil.
4. Stir in the jasmine rice and reduce heat to low. Cover and simmer for 15 minutes.
5. Add the shrimp and dried thyme, and cook for an additional 5-7 minutes, or until the shrimp are pink and opaque and the rice is tender.
6. Garnish with fresh parsley before serving.

Nutrition Info (Per Serving):

- Calories: 250
- Protein: 25g
- Carbohydrates: 28g
- Dietary Fiber: 2g
- Sugars: 3g
- Total Fat: 6g
- Saturated Fat: 1g
- Sodium: 200mg

Serves:

- **4 servings**

Cooking Time:

- **Total: 30 minutes**

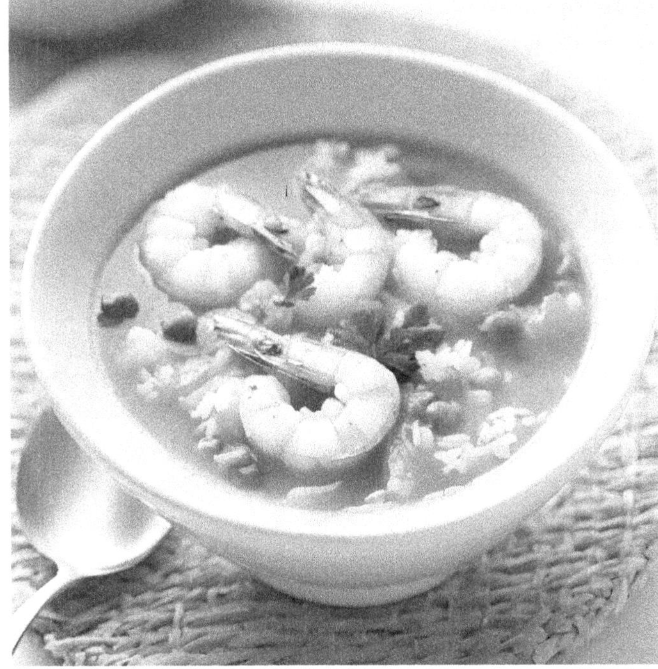

5. Grilled Trout with Olive Oil

Ingredients:

- 4 trout fillets (about 6 ounces each)
- 2 tablespoons of olive oil
- 1 teaspoon of dried thyme
- 1 teaspoon of dried rosemary
- 1 lemon, sliced (if tolerated)
- Fresh parsley for garnish

Instructions:

1. Preheat the grill to medium-high heat.
2. Brush the trout fillets with olive oil and sprinkle with dried thyme and rosemary.
3. Place the trout fillets on the grill, skin side down.
4. Grill for 4-5 minutes on each side, or until the fish is cooked through and flakes easily with a fork.
5. Garnish with lemon slices (if tolerated) and fresh parsley before serving.

Nutrition Info (Per Serving):

- Calories: 250
- Protein: 28g
- Carbohydrates: 1g
- Dietary Fiber: 0g
- Sugars: 0g
- Total Fat: 14g
- Saturated Fat: 2g
- Sodium: 70mg

Serves:

- **4 servings**

Cooking Time:

- **Total: 15 minutes**

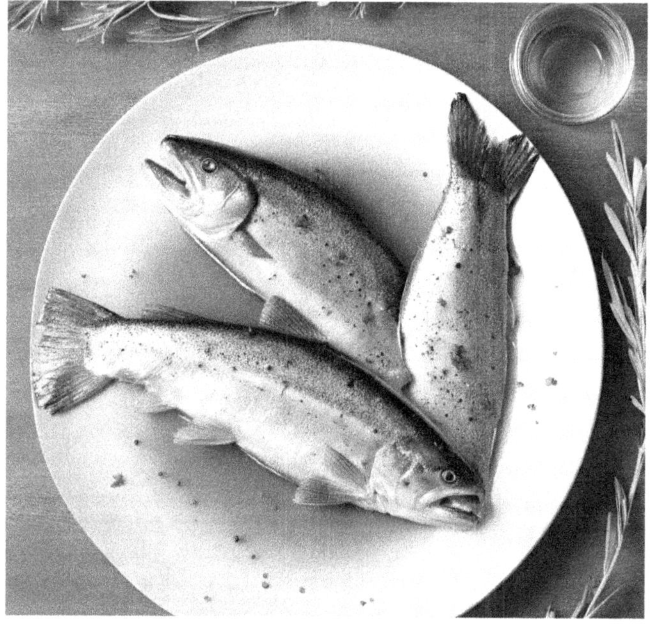

6. Scallops with Ginger

Ingredients:

- 1 pound of scallops
- 1 tablespoon of olive oil
- 1 tablespoon of fresh ginger, grated
- 1/4 cup of low-sodium chicken or vegetable broth
- Fresh cilantro for garnish

Instructions:

1. Rinse the scallops and pat them dry with paper towels.
2. Heat the olive oil in a large skillet over medium heat.
3. Add the grated ginger and cook for 1-2 minutes until fragrant.
4. Add the scallops to the skillet and cook for 2-3 minutes on each side until they are opaque and slightly golden.
5. Pour in the broth and cook for an additional 2 minutes.
6. Garnish with fresh cilantro before serving.

Nutrition Info (Per Serving):

- Calories: 180
- Protein: 24g
- Carbohydrates: 2g
- Dietary Fiber: 0g
- Sugars: 0g
- Total Fat: 7g
- Saturated Fat: 1g
- Sodium: 200mg

Serves:

- **4 servings**

Cooking Time:

- **Total: 10 minutes**

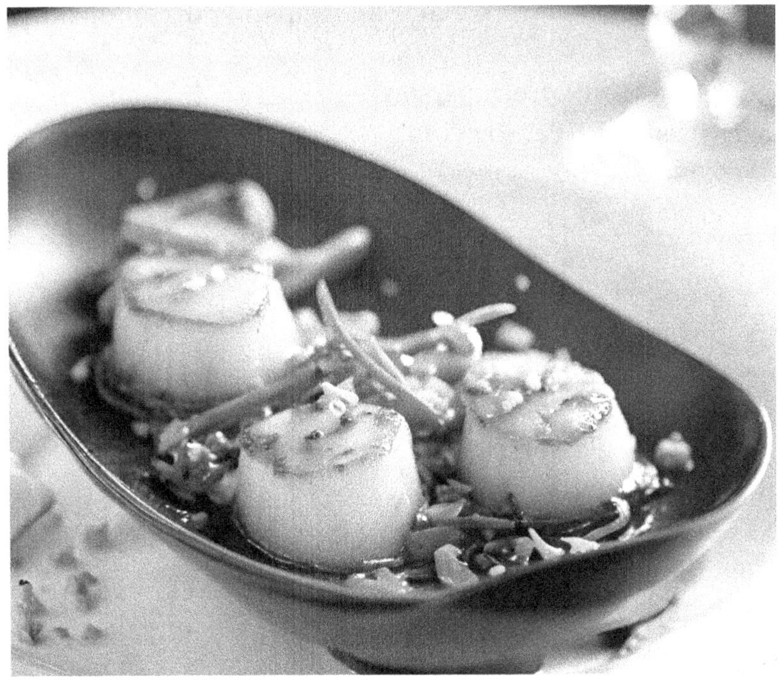

7. Clam Chowder

Ingredients:

- 2 cups of chopped clams (fresh or canned, drained)
- 4 cups of low-sodium chicken broth
- 2 medium potatoes, diced
- 2 celery stalks, diced
- 2 medium carrots, diced
- 1 cup of unsweetened almond milk
- 2 tablespoons of olive oil
- 1 teaspoon of dried thyme
- 1 bay leaf
- Fresh parsley for garnish

Instructions:

1. In a large pot, heat the olive oil over medium heat.
2. Add the diced potatoes, celery, and carrots, and cook for 5-7 minutes until slightly softened.
3. Add the chicken broth, thyme, and bay leaf to the pot. Bring to a boil.
4. Reduce heat to low and simmer for 15 minutes, or until the vegetables are tender.
5. Stir in the chopped clams and almond milk, and cook for an additional 5 minutes.
6. Remove the bay leaf before serving.
7. Garnish with fresh parsley.

Nutrition Info (Per Serving):

- Calories: 200
- Protein: 12g
- Carbohydrates: 20g
- Dietary Fiber: 3g
- Sugars: 4g
- Total Fat: 8g
- Saturated Fat: 1g
- Sodium: 250mg

Serves:

- **4 servings**

Cooking Time:

- **Total: 30 minutes**

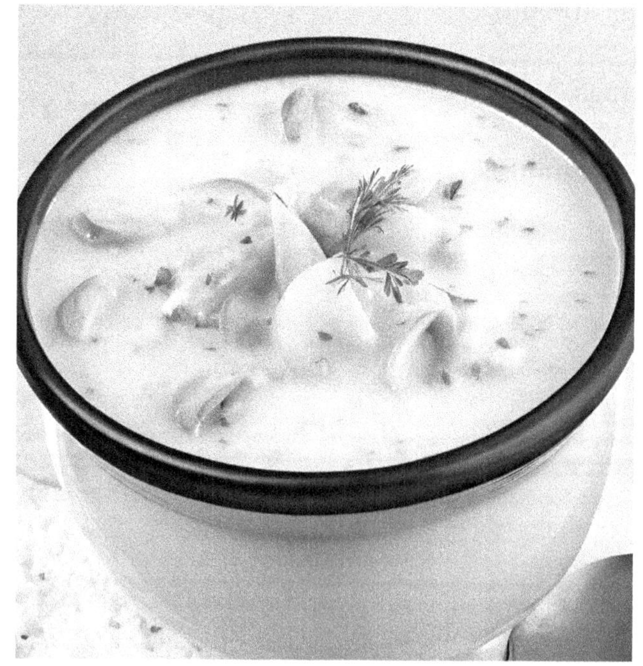

8. Mackerel in Foil

Ingredients:

- 4 mackerel fillets (about 6 ounces each)
- 2 tablespoons of olive oil
- 1 teaspoon of dried dill
- 1 teaspoon of dried parsley
- 1 lemon, thinly sliced (if tolerated)
- Fresh dill for garnish

Instructions:

1. Preheat the oven to 375°F (190°C).
2. Place each mackerel fillet on a piece of aluminum foil.
3. Brush the fillets with olive oil and sprinkle with dried dill and parsley.
4. Add a few lemon slices on top of each fillet (if tolerated).
5. Fold the foil over the fish to create a sealed packet.
6. Place the foil packets on a baking sheet and bake for 20-25 minutes, or until the fish is cooked through and flakes easily with a fork.
7. Garnish with fresh dill before serving.

Nutrition Info (Per Serving):

- Calories: 300
- Protein: 25g
- Carbohydrates: 2g
- Dietary Fiber: 0g
- Sugars: 0g
- Total Fat: 20g
- Saturated Fat: 4g
- Sodium: 80mg

Serves:

- **4 servings**

Cooking Time:

- **Total: 30 minutes**

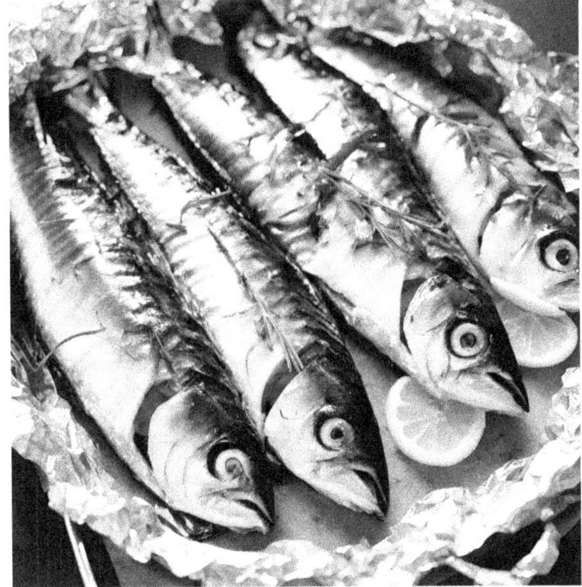

9. Sea Bass with Parsley Sauce

Ingredients:

- 4 sea bass fillets (about 6 ounces each)
- 2 tablespoons of olive oil
- 1/4 cup of fresh parsley, finely chopped
- 1/2 cup of low-sodium chicken or vegetable broth
- 1 tablespoon of unsalted butter
- Fresh parsley for garnish

Instructions:

1. Preheat the oven to 375°F (190°C).
2. Brush the sea bass fillets with olive oil and place them in a baking dish.
3. Bake for 15-20 minutes, or until the fish is opaque and flakes easily with a fork.
4. In a small saucepan, heat the broth and butter over medium heat until the butter is melted.
5. Stir in the chopped parsley and cook for 2-3 minutes.
6. Serve the sea bass with the parsley sauce and garnish with fresh parsley.

Nutrition Info (Per Serving):

- Calories: 250
- Protein: 28g
- Carbohydrates: 1g
- Dietary Fiber: 0g
- Sugars: 0g
- Total Fat: 14g
- Saturated Fat: 4g
- Sodium: 150mg

Serves:

- **4 servings**

Cooking Time:

- **Total: 25 minutes**

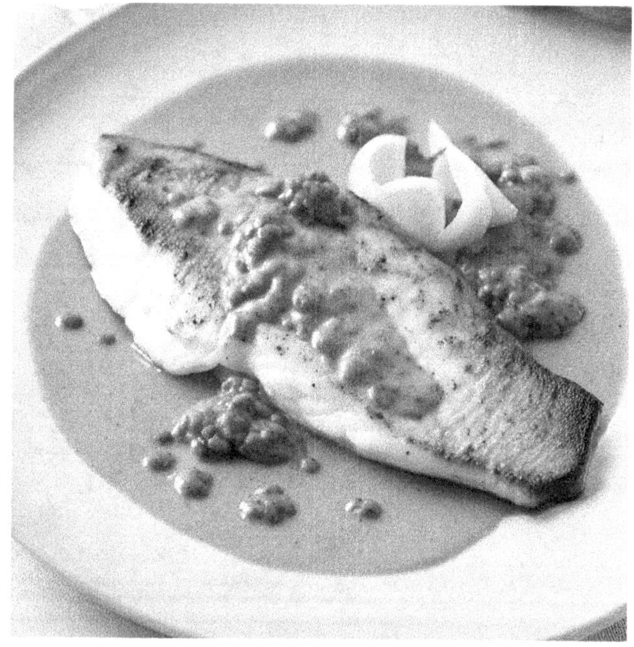

10. Broiled Haddock

Ingredients:

- 4 haddock fillets (about 6 ounces each)
- 2 tablespoons of olive oil
- 1 teaspoon of dried thyme
- 1 teaspoon of dried rosemary
- Fresh parsley for garnish

Instructions:

1. Preheat the broiler to high.
2. Brush the haddock fillets with olive oil and sprinkle with dried thyme and rosemary.
3. Place the fillets on a broiler pan and broil for 4-5 minutes on each side, or until the fish is opaque and flakes easily with a fork.
4. Garnish with fresh parsley before serving.

Nutrition Info (Per Serving):

- Calories: 210
- Protein: 30g
- Carbohydrates: 0g
- Dietary Fiber: 0g
- Sugars: 0g
- Total Fat: 9g
- Saturated Fat: 1g
- Sodium: 80mg

Serves:

- **4 servings**

Cooking Time:

- **Total: 10 minutes**

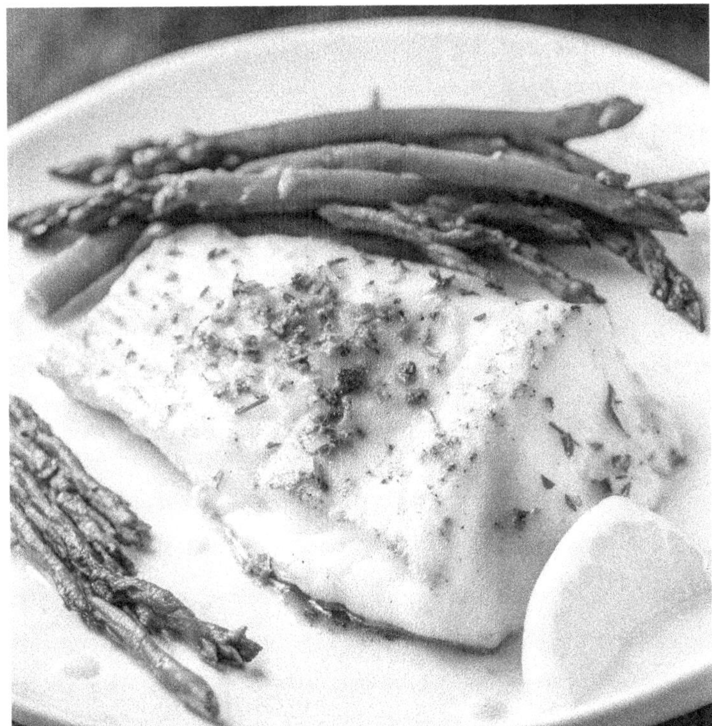

11. Halibut with Mint Peas

Ingredients:

- 4 halibut fillets (about 6 ounces each)
- 2 tablespoons of olive oil
- 1 cup of peas (fresh or frozen)
- 1/4 cup of fresh mint leaves, chopped
- 1/2 cup of low-sodium vegetable broth

Instructions:

1. Preheat the oven to 375°F (190°C).
2. Brush the halibut fillets with olive oil and place them in a baking dish.
3. Bake for 15-20 minutes, or until the fish is opaque and flakes easily with a fork.
4. In a small saucepan, bring the vegetable broth to a simmer.
5. Add the peas and cook for 3-4 minutes until tender.
6. Stir in the chopped mint leaves and cook for an additional minute.
7. Serve the halibut with the mint peas.

Nutrition Info (Per Serving):

- Calories: 220
- Protein: 28g
- Carbohydrates: 7g
- Dietary Fiber: 2g
- Sugars: 3g
- Total Fat: 9g
- Saturated Fat: 1g
- Sodium: 100mg

Serves:

- 4 servings

Cooking Time:

- **Total: 25 minutes**

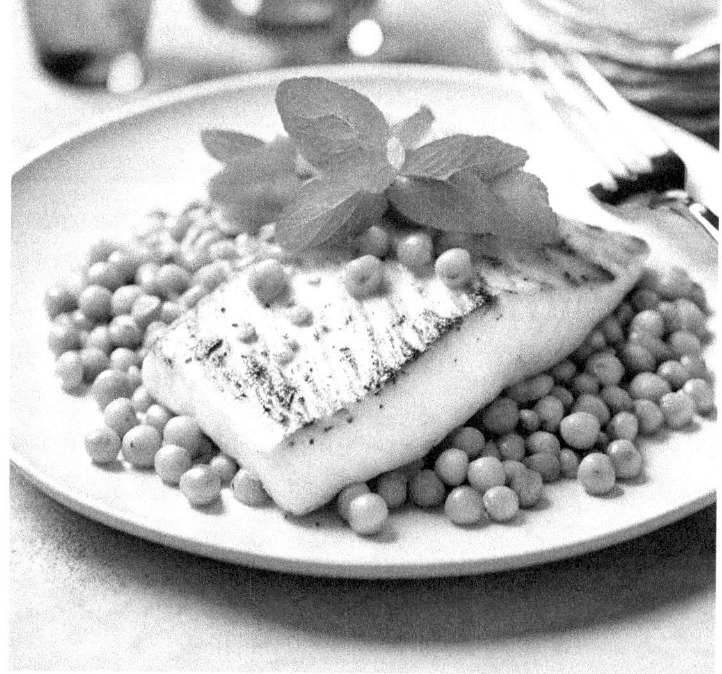

12. Sole Meunière

Ingredients:

- 4 sole fillets (about 6 ounces each)
- 1/4 cup of whole wheat flour
- 2 tablespoons of olive oil
- 2 tablespoons of unsalted butter
- 1/4 cup of fresh parsley, chopped
- Fresh lemon wedges (if tolerated)

Instructions:

1. Dredge the sole fillets in the whole wheat flour, shaking off any excess.
2. Heat the olive oil and 1 tablespoon of butter in a large skillet over medium heat.
3. Add the sole fillets to the skillet and cook for 2-3 minutes on each side, until golden brown and cooked through.
4. Remove the fillets from the skillet and place on a serving platter.
5. Add the remaining butter to the skillet and melt, stirring in the chopped parsley.
6. Pour the parsley butter over the sole fillets.
7. Serve with fresh lemon wedges (if tolerated).

Nutrition Info (Per Serving):

- Calories: 250
- Protein: 30g
- Carbohydrates: 4g
- Dietary Fiber: 1g
- Sugars: 0g
- Total Fat: 12g
- Saturated Fat: 4g
- Sodium: 150mg

Serves:

- **4 servings**

Cooking Time:

- **Total: 15 minutes**

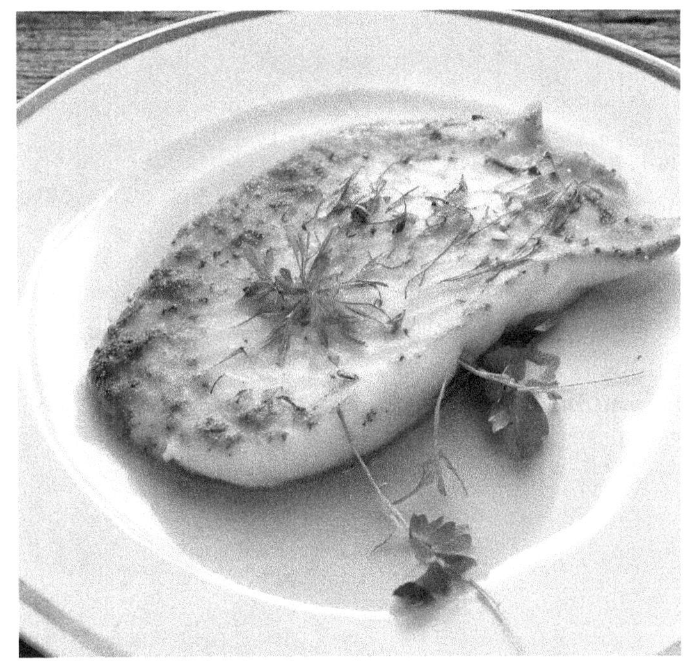

13. Oyster Stew

Ingredients:

- 1 pint of fresh oysters, with liquid
- 4 cups of low-sodium chicken broth
- 1 cup of unsweetened almond milk
- 2 medium potatoes, peeled and diced
- 2 celery stalks, diced
- 2 tablespoons of unsalted butter
- 1 teaspoon of dried thyme
- Fresh parsley for garnish

Instructions:

1. In a large pot, melt the butter over medium heat.
2. Add the diced potatoes and celery, and cook for 5-7 minutes until slightly softened.
3. Add the chicken broth and thyme, and bring to a boil.
4. Reduce heat to low and simmer for 15 minutes, or until the potatoes are tender.
5. Stir in the oysters with their liquid and almond milk, and cook for an additional 5 minutes until the oysters are cooked through.
6. Garnish with fresh parsley before serving.

Nutrition Info (Per Serving):

- Calories: 200
- Protein: 10g
- Carbohydrates: 20g
- Dietary Fiber: 2g
- Sugars: 4g
- Total Fat: 8g
- Saturated Fat: 3g
- Sodium: 200mg

Serves:

- **4 servings**

Cooking Time:

- **Total: 30 minute**

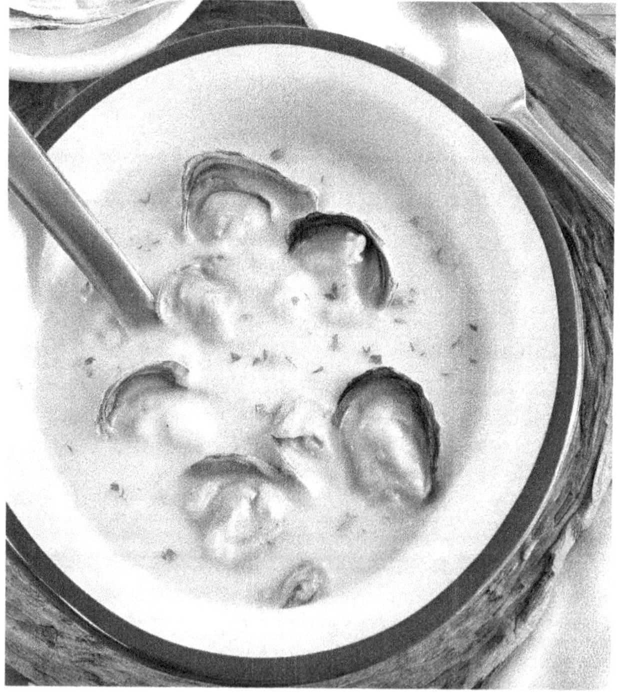

14. Grouper with Mango Salsa

Ingredients:

- 4 grouper fillets (about 6 ounces each)
- 2 tablespoons of olive oil
- 1 ripe mango, peeled and diced
- 1/2 cup of diced cucumber
- 1/4 cup of diced red onion (if tolerated)
- 1/4 cup of fresh cilantro, chopped
- Juice of 1 lime (if tolerated)

Instructions:

1. Preheat the grill to medium-high heat.
2. Brush the grouper fillets with olive oil.
3. Grill the fillets for 4-5 minutes on each side, or until the fish is opaque and flakes easily with a fork.
4. In a bowl, combine the mango, cucumber, red onion (if tolerated), cilantro, and lime juice (if tolerated).
5. Serve the grilled grouper topped with the mango salsa.

Nutrition Info (Per Serving):

- Calories: 260
- Protein: 28g
- Carbohydrates: 10g
- Dietary Fiber: 2g
- Sugars: 8g
- Total Fat: 12g
- Saturated Fat: 2g
- Sodium: 80mg

Serves:

- **4 servings**

Cooking Time:

- **Total: 20 minutes**

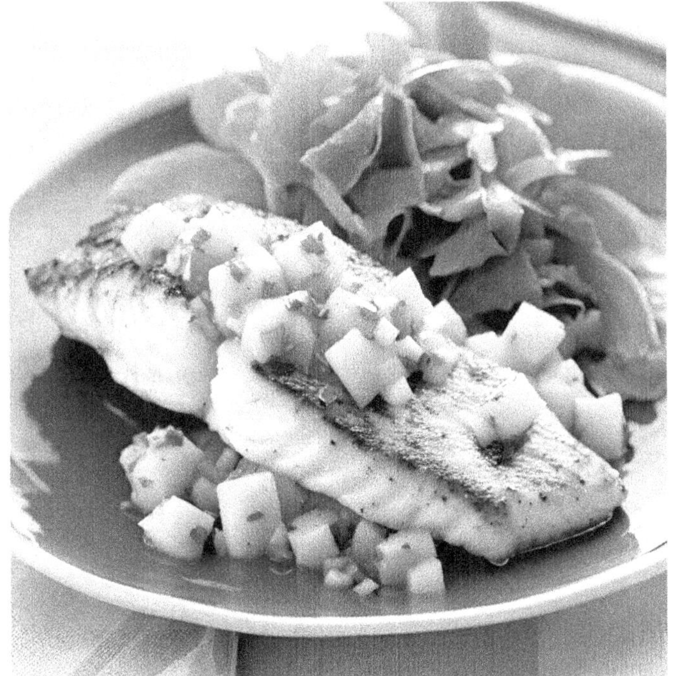

15. Salmon Patties

Ingredients:

- 1 pound of cooked salmon, flaked
- 1/2 cup of whole wheat breadcrumbs
- 1/4 cup of plain yogurt (dairy or soy)
- 1 large egg, beaten
- 2 tablespoons of fresh dill, chopped
- 1 tablespoon of olive oil

Instructions:

1. In a large bowl, combine the flaked salmon, breadcrumbs, yogurt, beaten egg, and fresh dill.
2. Mix well and form the mixture into 4 patties.
3. Heat the olive oil in a large skillet over medium heat.
4. Cook the patties for 3-4 minutes on each side, until golden brown and heated through.
5. Serve warm.

Nutrition Info (Per Serving):

- Calories: 300
- Protein: 28g
- Carbohydrates: 10g
- Dietary Fiber: 2g
- Sugars: 1g
- Total Fat: 16g
- Saturated Fat: 3g
- Sodium: 200mg

Serves:

- **4 servings**

Cooking Time:

- **Total: 20 minutes**

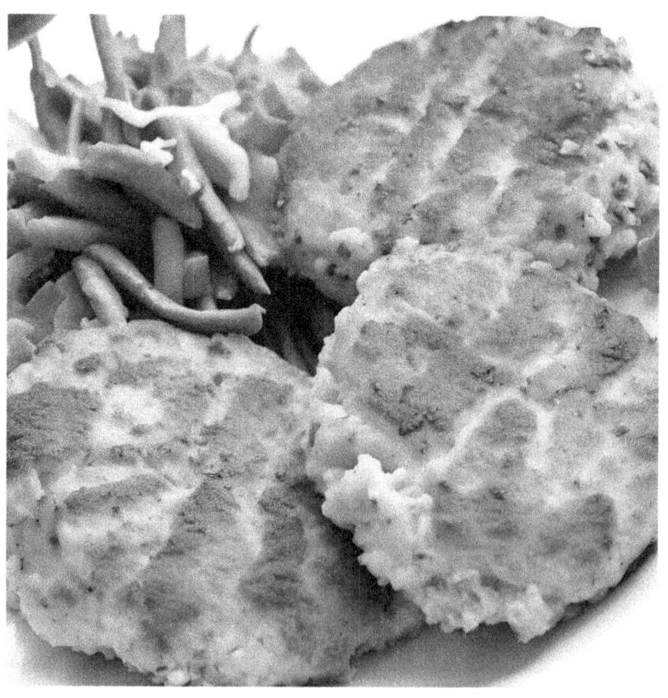

16. Trout Almondine

Ingredients:

- 4 trout fillets (about 6 ounces each)
- 1/4 cup of whole wheat flour
- 2 tablespoons of olive oil
- 1/4 cup of sliced almonds
- 2 tablespoons of unsalted butter
- Juice of 1 lemon (if tolerated)
- Fresh parsley for garnish

Instructions:

1. Dredge the trout fillets in the whole wheat flour, shaking off any excess.
2. Heat the olive oil in a large skillet over medium heat.
3. Add the trout fillets and cook for 2-3 minutes on each side, until golden brown and cooked through.
4. Remove the fillets from the skillet and place on a serving platter.
5. Add the butter to the skillet and melt, then stir in the sliced almonds and cook for 2-3 minutes until golden brown.
6. Drizzle the lemon juice (if tolerated) over the trout and top with the almond mixture.
7. Garnish with fresh parsley before serving.

Nutrition Info (Per Serving):

- Calories: 350
- Protein: 30g
- Carbohydrates: 6g
- Dietary Fiber: 2g
- Sugars: 0g
- Total Fat: 24g
- Saturated Fat: 8g
- Sodium: 120mg

Serves:

- **4 servings**

Cooking Time:

- **Total: 20 minutes**

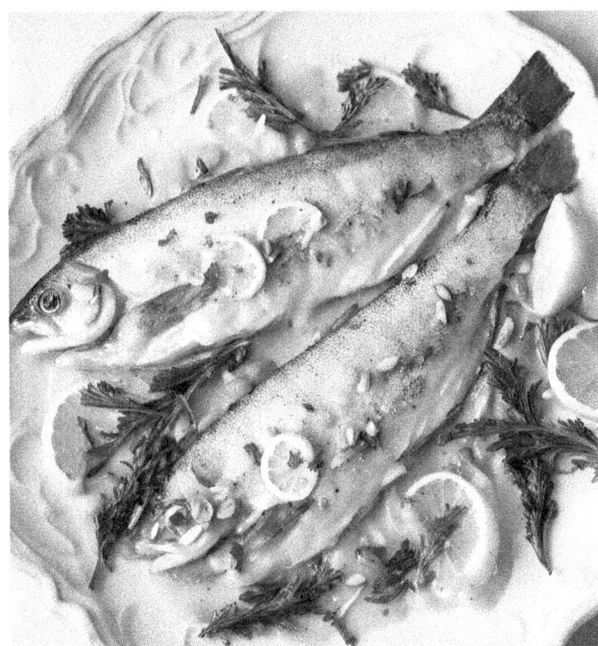

17. Catfish Soup

Ingredients:

- 1 pound of catfish fillets, cut into chunks
- 4 cups of low-sodium chicken broth
- 2 medium potatoes, peeled and diced
- 2 celery stalks, diced
- 2 medium carrots, diced
- 1 tablespoon of olive oil
- 1 teaspoon of dried thyme
- Fresh parsley for garnish

Instructions:

1. In a large pot, heat the olive oil over medium heat.
2. Add the diced potatoes, celery, and carrots, and cook for 5-7 minutes until slightly softened.
3. Add the chicken broth and thyme, and bring to a boil.
4. Reduce heat to low and simmer for 15 minutes, or until the vegetables are tender.
5. Stir in the catfish chunks and cook for an additional 5-7 minutes until the fish is opaque and cooked through.
6. Garnish with fresh parsley before serving.

Nutrition Info (Per Serving):

- Calories: 200
- Protein: 20g
- Carbohydrates: 18g
- Dietary Fiber: 3g
- Sugars: 4g
- Total Fat: 6g
- Saturated Fat: 1g
- Sodium: 180mg

Serves:

- **4 servings**

Cooking Time:

- **Total: 30 minutes**

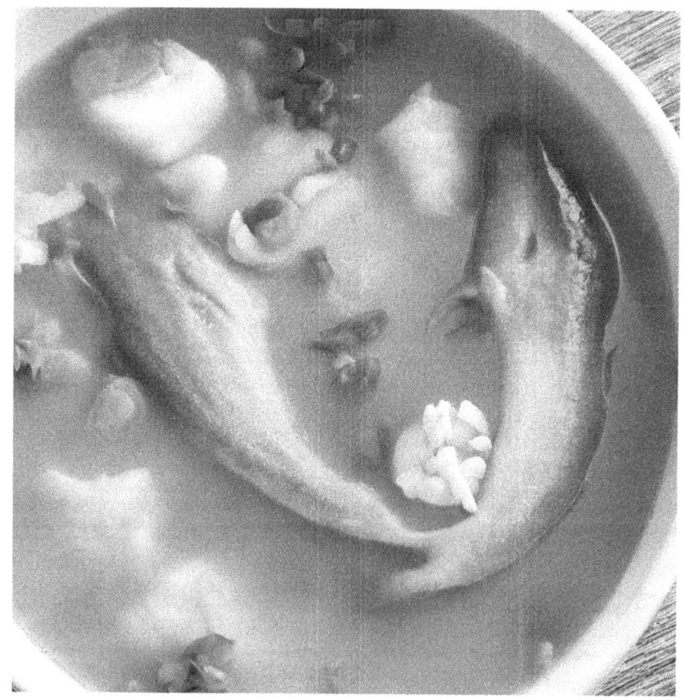

18. Barramundi with Basil

Ingredients:

- 4 barramundi fillets (about 6 ounces each)
- 2 tablespoons of olive oil
- 1/2 cup of fresh basil leaves, chopped
- 1/2 cup of low-sodium vegetable broth
- 1 tablespoon of unsalted butter
- Fresh basil for garnish

Instructions:

1. Preheat the oven to 375°F (190°C).
2. Brush the barramundi fillets with olive oil and place them in a baking dish.
3. Bake for 15-20 minutes, or until the fish is opaque and flakes easily with a fork.
4. In a small saucepan, heat the broth and butter over medium heat until the butter is melted.
5. Stir in the chopped basil and cook for 2-3 minutes.
6. Serve the barramundi with the basil sauce and garnish with fresh basil.

Nutrition Info (Per Serving):

- Calories: 240
- Protein: 28g
- Carbohydrates: 2g
- Dietary Fiber: 0g
- Sugars: 0g
- Total Fat: 14g
- Saturated Fat: 4g
- Sodium: 150mg

Serves:

- **4 servings**

Cooking Time:

- **Total: 25 minutes**

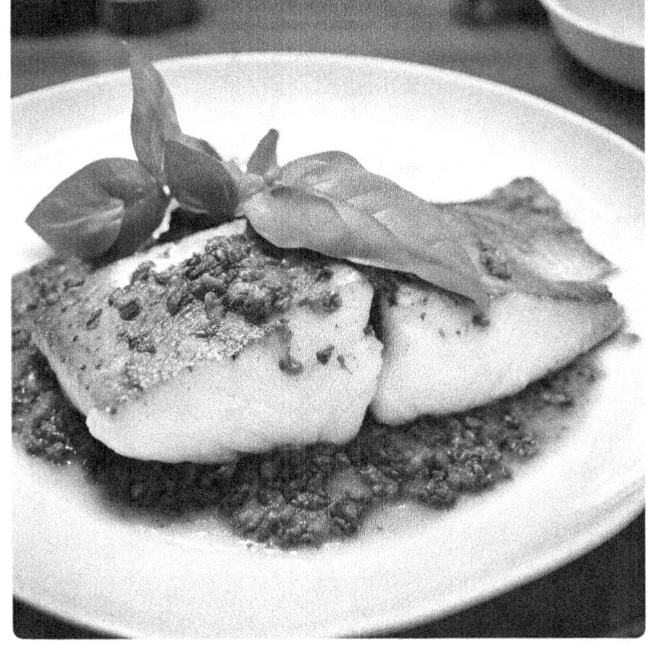

19. Fish Congee

Ingredients:

- 1 cup of jasmine rice
- 8 cups of low-sodium chicken or vegetable broth
- 1 pound of white fish fillets (such as cod or haddock), cut into chunks
- 2 tablespoons of fresh ginger, julienned
- 2 tablespoons of olive oil
- Fresh cilantro for garnish

Instructions:

1. Rinse the jasmine rice under cold water until the water runs clear.
2. In a large pot, bring the broth to a boil.
3. Add the rice to the pot and reduce heat to low. Simmer for about 1 hour, stirring occasionally, until the rice has broken down and the congee has thickened.
4. In a skillet, heat the olive oil over medium heat and sauté the ginger until fragrant.
5. Add the ginger and white fish chunks to the congee. Cook for an additional 10 minutes until the fish is cooked through and flakes easily.
6. Serve hot, garnished with fresh cilantro.

Nutrition Info (Per Serving):

- Calories: 250
- Protein: 20g
- Carbohydrates: 32g
- Dietary Fiber: 1g
- Sugars: 1g
- Total Fat: 6g
- Saturated Fat: 1g
- Sodium: 200mg

Serves:

- **4 servings**

Cooking Time:

- **Total: 70 minutes**

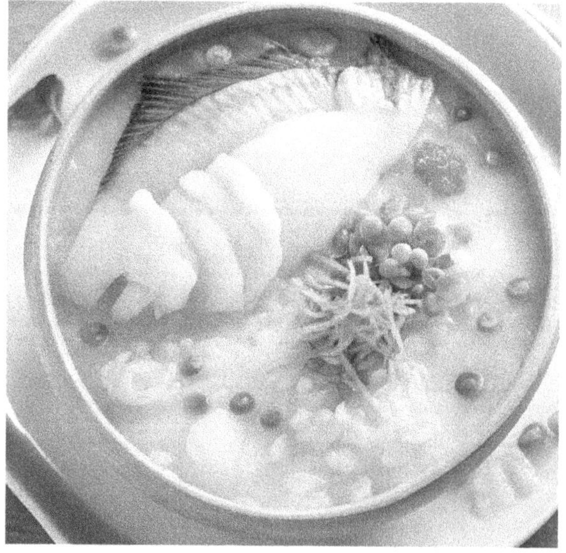

20. Sardines with Herbs

Ingredients:

- 4 fresh sardine fillets
- 2 tablespoons of olive oil
- 1 teaspoon of dried thyme
- 1 teaspoon of dried rosemary
- 1 teaspoon of dried parsley
- Fresh lemon wedges (if tolerated)

Instructions:

1. Preheat the oven to 400°F (200°C).
2. Place the sardine fillets on a baking sheet lined with parchment paper.
3. Brush the fillets with olive oil and sprinkle with dried thyme, rosemary, and parsley.
4. Bake for 10-12 minutes, or until the sardines are cooked through and the flesh is firm.
5. Serve with fresh lemon wedges (if tolerated).

Nutrition Info (Per Serving):

- Calories: 180
- Protein: 22g
- Carbohydrates: 1g
- Dietary Fiber: 0g
- Sugars: 0g
- Total Fat: 10g
- Saturated Fat: 2g
- Sodium: 150mg

Serves:

- 2 servings

Cooking Time:

- **Total: 15 minutes**

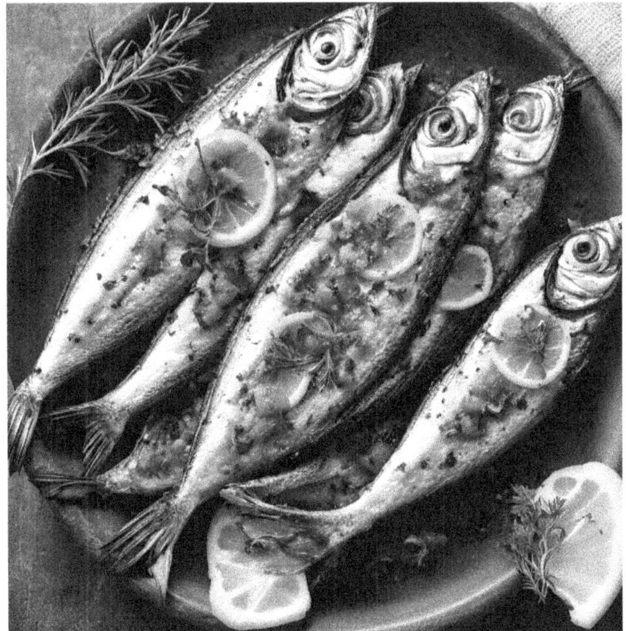

21. Shrimp Pasta

Ingredients:

- 8 ounces of whole wheat pasta
- 1 pound of shrimp, peeled and deveined
- 2 tablespoons of olive oil
- 1 cup of low-sodium vegetable broth
- 1/4 cup of fresh basil, chopped
- 1/4 cup of grated Parmesan cheese (optional)
- Fresh basil leaves for garnish

Instructions:

1. Cook the pasta according to package instructions. Drain and set aside.
2. In a large skillet, heat the olive oil over medium heat.
3. Add the shrimp and cook for 3-4 minutes, until pink and opaque.
4. Add the vegetable broth and fresh basil to the skillet, and simmer for an additional 2 minutes.
5. Toss the cooked pasta with the shrimp and broth mixture.
6. Serve topped with grated Parmesan cheese (if using) and garnished with fresh basil leaves.

Nutrition Info (Per Serving):

- Calories: 350
- Protein: 30g
- Carbohydrates: 45g
- Dietary Fiber: 8g
- Sugars: 2g
- Total Fat: 8g
- Saturated Fat: 2g
- Sodium: 200mg

Serves:

- 4 servings

Cooking Time:

- Total: 20 minutes

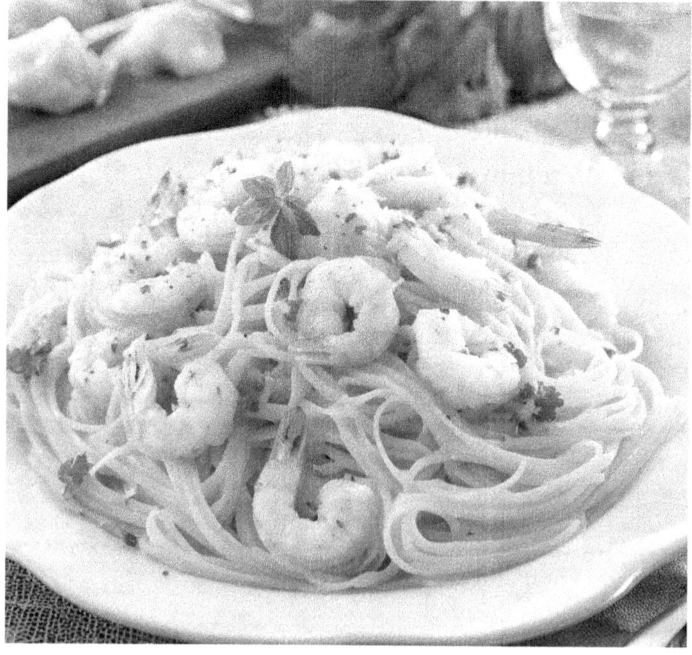

22. Baked Snapper with Rosemary

Ingredients:

- 4 snapper fillets (about 6 ounces each)
- 2 tablespoons of olive oil
- 1 teaspoon of dried rosemary
- 1/2 cup of low-sodium chicken or vegetable broth
- Fresh parsley for garnish

Instructions:

1. Preheat the oven to 375°F (190°C).
2. Brush the snapper fillets with olive oil and sprinkle with dried rosemary.
3. Place the fillets in a baking dish and pour the broth around them.
4. Bake for 15-20 minutes, or until the fish is opaque and flakes easily with a fork.
5. Garnish with fresh parsley before serving.

Nutrition Info (Per Serving):

- Calories: 240
- Protein: 28g
- Carbohydrates: 1g
- Dietary Fiber: 0g
- Sugars: 0g
- Total Fat: 12g
- Saturated Fat: 2g
- Sodium: 100mg

Serves:

- **4 servings**

Cooking Time:

- **Total: 25 minutes**

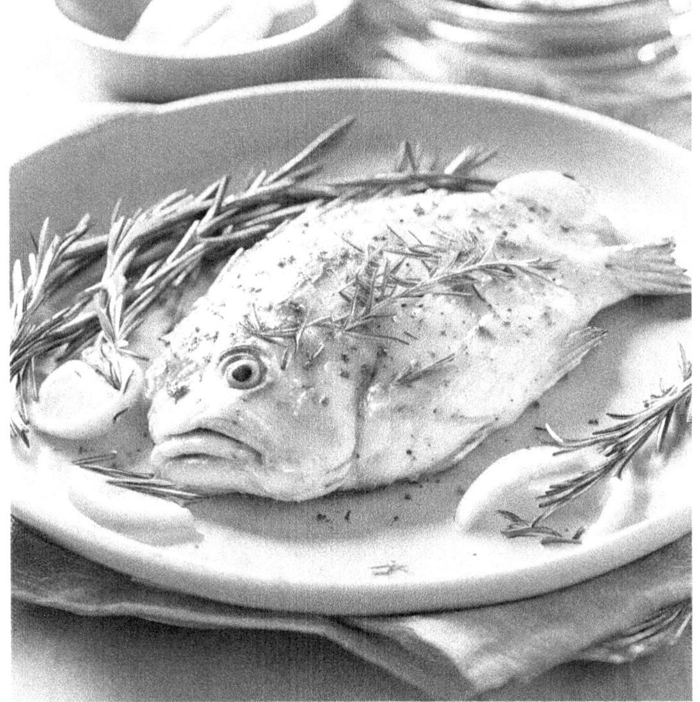

23. Fish Fillet with Carrot Puree

Ingredients:

- 4 white fish fillets (such as cod or haddock)
- 2 tablespoons of olive oil
- 1 pound of carrots, peeled and chopped
- 1/4 cup of unsweetened almond milk
- 1 teaspoon of dried thyme
- Fresh parsley for garnish

Instructions:

1. Preheat the oven to 375°F (190°C).
2. Brush the fish fillets with olive oil and place them on a baking sheet.
3. Bake for 15-20 minutes, or until the fish is opaque and flakes easily with a fork.
4. Meanwhile, in a large pot, bring water to a boil and add the chopped carrots. Cook for 10-15 minutes until tender.
5. Drain the carrots and transfer to a blender. Add the almond milk and dried thyme, and blend until smooth.
6. Serve the fish fillets with the carrot puree and garnish with fresh parsley.

Nutrition Info (Per Serving):

- Calories: 220
- Protein: 25g
- Carbohydrates: 20g
- Dietary Fiber: 5g
- Sugars: 10g
- Total Fat: 6g
- Saturated Fat: 1g
- Sodium: 100mg

Serves:

- **4 servings**

Cooking Time:

- **Total: 30 minutes**

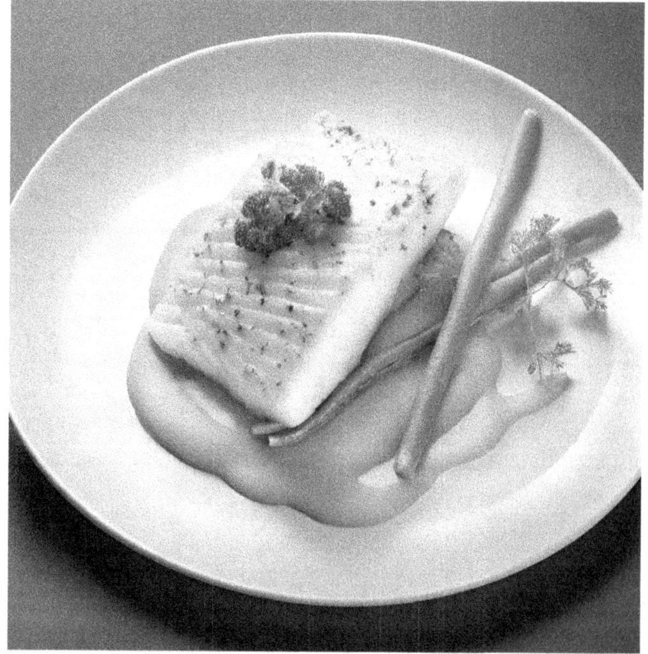

24. Scallop Risotto

Ingredients:

- 1 pound of scallops
- 1 1/2 cups of arborio rice
- 4 cups of low-sodium chicken or vegetable broth
- 1 cup of unsweetened almond milk
- 2 tablespoons of olive oil
- 1/2 cup of grated Parmesan cheese (optional)
- 1/4 cup of fresh parsley, chopped
- 1 teaspoon of dried thyme

Instructions:

1. In a medium saucepan, heat the broth and keep it warm over low heat.
2. In a large skillet, heat 1 tablespoon of olive oil over medium heat.
3. Add the arborio rice and cook for 2-3 minutes, stirring frequently, until the rice is lightly toasted.
4. Begin adding the warm broth, one ladle at a time, stirring continuously and allowing each addition to be absorbed before adding more. Continue this process for about 20 minutes, or until the rice is creamy and cooked through.
5. Meanwhile, in another skillet, heat the remaining olive oil over medium heat. Add the scallops and cook for 2-3 minutes on each side, until they are opaque and slightly golden.
6. Once the risotto is done, stir in the almond milk, Parmesan cheese (if using), and dried thyme.
7. Serve the risotto topped with scallops and garnished with fresh parsley.

Nutrition Info (Per Serving):

- Calories: 400
- Protein: 30g
- Carbohydrates: 45g
- Dietary Fiber: 2g
- Sugars: 2g
- Total Fat: 12g
- Saturated Fat: 2g
- Sodium: 300mg

Serves:

- **4 servings**

Cooking Time:

- **Total: 30 minutes**

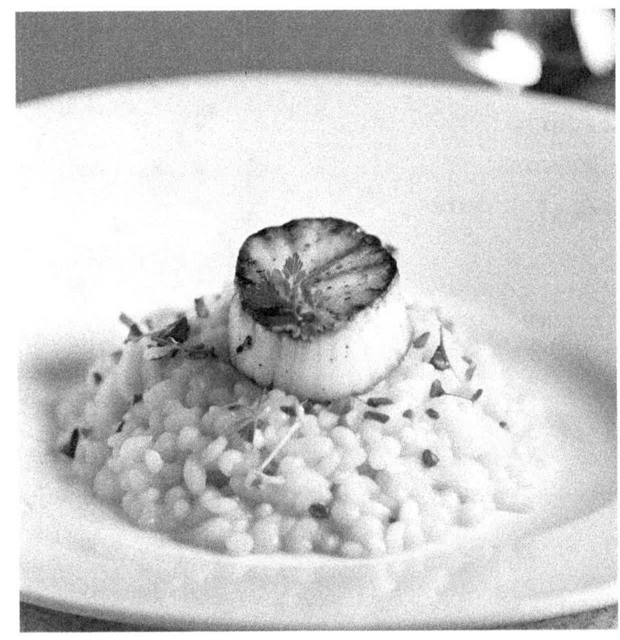

25. Pike in Parchment

Ingredients:

- 4 pike fillets (about 6 ounces each)
- 2 tablespoons of olive oil
- 1 lemon, thinly sliced (if tolerated)
- 1 teaspoon of dried thyme
- 1 teaspoon of dried rosemary
- Fresh parsley for garnish

Instructions:

1. Preheat the oven to 375°F (190°C).
2. Place each pike fillet on a piece of parchment paper.
3. Brush the fillets with olive oil and sprinkle with dried thyme and rosemary.
4. Add a few lemon slices on top of each fillet (if tolerated).
5. Fold the parchment paper over the fish to create a sealed packet.
6. Place the packets on a baking sheet and bake for 20-25 minutes, or until the fish is opaque and flakes easily with a fork.
7. Garnish with fresh parsley before serving.

Nutrition Info (Per Serving):

- Calories: 220
- Protein: 30g
- Carbohydrates: 1g
- Dietary Fiber: 0g
- Sugars: 0g
- Total Fat: 10g
- Saturated Fat: 2g
- Sodium: 80mg

Serves:

- **4 servings**

Cooking Time:

- **Total: 25 minutes**

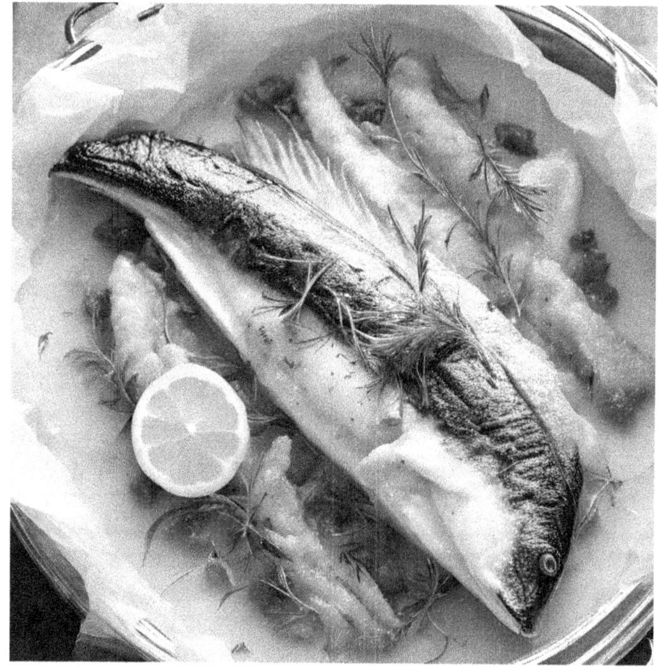

26. Salmon and Spinach Quiche

Ingredients:

- 1 premade whole wheat pie crust
- 1 cup of cooked salmon, flaked
- 1 cup of fresh spinach, chopped
- 4 large eggs
- 1 cup of unsweetened almond milk
- 1/2 cup of grated low-fat cheese (optional)
- 1 teaspoon of dried dill

Instructions:

1. Preheat the oven to 375°F (190°C).
2. Place the pie crust in a pie dish and set aside.
3. In a large bowl, whisk together the eggs, almond milk, and dried dill.
4. Spread the flaked salmon and chopped spinach evenly in the pie crust.
5. Pour the egg mixture over the salmon and spinach.
6. Sprinkle with grated cheese (if using).
7. Bake for 35-40 minutes, or until the quiche is set and lightly golden.
8. Let cool slightly before slicing and serving.

Nutrition Info (Per Serving):

- Calories: 250
- Protein: 20g
- Carbohydrates: 15g
- Dietary Fiber: 2g
- Sugars: 1g
- Total Fat: 14g
- Saturated Fat: 4g
- Sodium: 200mg

Serves:

- **6 servings**

Cooking Time:

- **Total: 45 minutes**

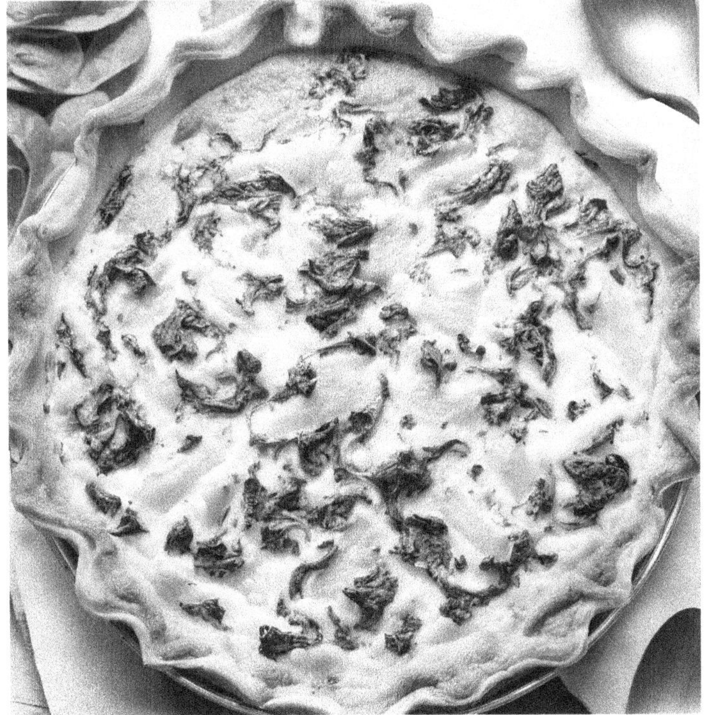

27. Cod with Parsnip Mash

Ingredients:

- 4 cod fillets (about 6 ounces each)
- 2 tablespoons of olive oil
- 1 pound of parsnips, peeled and chopped
- 1/2 cup of unsweetened almond milk
- 1 teaspoon of dried thyme
- Fresh parsley for garnish

Instructions:

1. Preheat the oven to 375°F (190°C).
2. Brush the cod fillets with olive oil and place them on a baking sheet.
3. Bake for 15-20 minutes, or until the fish is opaque and flakes easily with a fork.
4. Meanwhile, in a large pot, bring water to a boil and add the chopped parsnips. Cook for 10-15 minutes until tender.
5. Drain the parsnips and transfer to a blender. Add the almond milk and dried thyme, and blend until smooth.
6. Serve the cod fillets with the parsnip mash and garnish with fresh parsley.

Nutrition Info (Per Serving):

- Calories: 230
- Protein: 25g
- Carbohydrates: 20g
- Dietary Fiber: 5g
- Sugars: 5g
- Total Fat: 6g
- Saturated Fat: 1g
- Sodium: 100mg

Serves:

- **4 servings**

Cooking Time:

- **Total: 30 minutes**

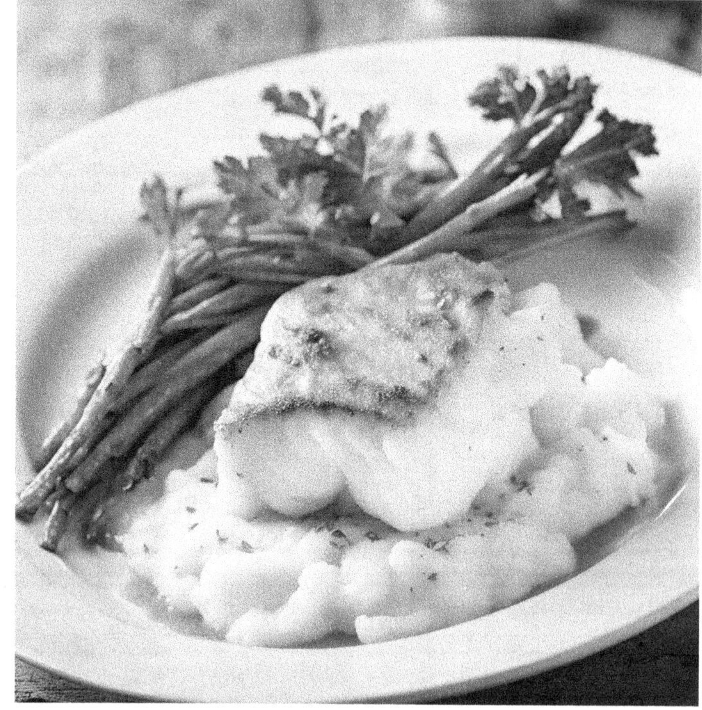

28. Rainbow Trout with Dill Yogurt

Ingredients:

- 4 rainbow trout fillets (about 6 ounces each)
- 2 tablespoons of olive oil
- 1/2 cup of plain yogurt (dairy or soy)
- 2 tablespoons of fresh dill, chopped
- 1 tablespoon of lemon juice (if tolerated)
- Fresh dill for garnish

Instructions:

1. Preheat the oven to 375°F (190°C).
2. Brush the trout fillets with olive oil and place them on a baking sheet.
3. Bake for 15-20 minutes, or until the fish is opaque and flakes easily with a fork.
4. In a small bowl, combine the yogurt, chopped dill, and lemon juice (if tolerated).
5. Serve the trout with the dill yogurt sauce and garnish with fresh dill.

Nutrition Info (Per Serving):

- Calories: 250
- Protein: 28g
- Carbohydrates: 3g
- Dietary Fiber: 0g
- Sugars: 1g
- Total Fat: 14g
- Saturated Fat: 3g
- Sodium: 120mg

Serves:

- **4 servings**

Cooking Time:

- **Total: 25 minutes**

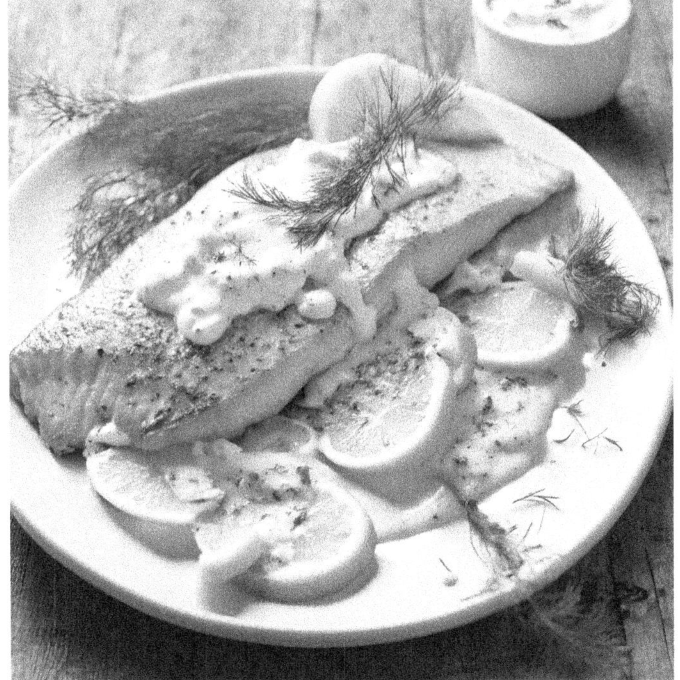

Poultry Recipes

1. Turkey Vegetable Soup

Ingredients:
- 1 pound of ground turkey
- 6 cups of low-sodium chicken or vegetable broth
- 2 medium carrots, diced
- 2 celery stalks, diced
- 1 medium potato, diced
- 1 cup of chopped spinach
- 1 tablespoon of olive oil
- 1 teaspoon of dried thyme
- Fresh parsley for garnish

Instructions:
1. In a large pot, heat the olive oil over medium heat.
2. Add the ground turkey and cook until browned, breaking it apart with a spoon.
3. Add the diced carrots, celery, and potato to the pot and cook for 5 minutes until slightly softened.
4. Pour in the broth and add the dried thyme. Bring to a boil.
5. Reduce heat to low and simmer for 20 minutes, or until the vegetables are tender.
6. Stir in the chopped spinach and cook for an additional 5 minutes.
7. Serve hot, garnished with fresh parsley.

Nutrition Info (Per Serving):
- Calories: 220
- Protein: 24g
- Carbohydrates: 18g
- Dietary Fiber: 3g
- Sugars: 4g
- Total Fat: 7g
- Saturated Fat: 2g
- Sodium: 150mg

Serves:
- **6 servings**

Cooking Time:
- **Total: 35 minutes**

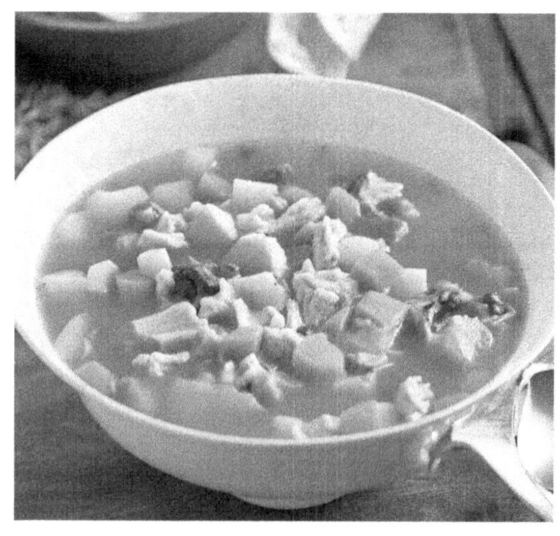

2. Baked Chicken with Barley

Ingredients:

- 4 boneless, skinless chicken breasts
- 1 cup of pearl barley
- 4 cups of low-sodium chicken broth
- 2 medium carrots, diced
- 2 celery stalks, diced
- 1 tablespoon of olive oil
- 1 teaspoon of dried rosemary
- 1 teaspoon of dried thyme
- Fresh parsley for garnish

Instructions:

1. Preheat the oven to 375°F (190°C).
2. In a large oven-safe pot or Dutch oven, heat the olive oil over medium heat.
3. Add the chicken breasts and cook for 5 minutes on each side, until browned.
4. Remove the chicken from the pot and set aside.
5. Add the diced carrots and celery to the pot and cook for 5 minutes until slightly softened.
6. Stir in the pearl barley and dried herbs.
7. Place the chicken breasts on top of the barley and vegetables.
8. Pour in the chicken broth and bring to a boil.
9. Cover the pot and transfer it to the oven. Bake for 45 minutes, or until the barley is tender and the chicken is cooked through.
10. Serve hot, garnished with fresh parsley.

Nutrition Info (Per Serving):

- Calories: 350
- Protein: 35g
- Carbohydrates: 40g
- Dietary Fiber: 7g
- Sugars: 4g
- Total Fat: 8g
- Saturated Fat: 2g
- Sodium: 200mg

Serves:

- **4 servings**

Cooking Time:

- **Total: 60 minutes**

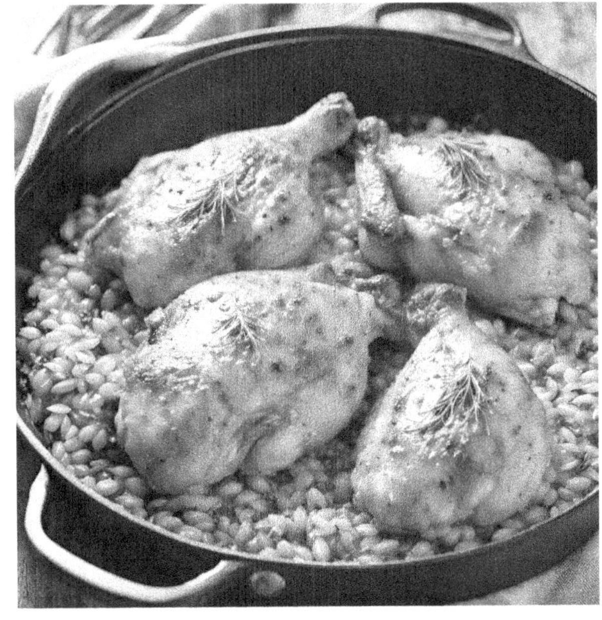

3. Turkey and Apple Stew

Ingredients:

- 1 pound of turkey breast, cubed
- 2 medium apples, peeled and chopped
- 2 medium carrots, diced
- 2 celery stalks, diced
- 4 cups of low-sodium chicken broth
- 1 tablespoon of olive oil
- 1 teaspoon of dried thyme
- 1 bay leaf
- Fresh parsley for garnish

Instructions:

1. In a large pot, heat the olive oil over medium heat.
2. Add the turkey cubes and cook until browned on all sides.
3. Add the diced carrots and celery and cook for 5 minutes until slightly softened.
4. Stir in the chopped apples and cook for another 3 minutes.
5. Pour in the chicken broth and add the dried thyme and bay leaf. Bring to a boil.
6. Reduce heat to low and simmer for 20-25 minutes, or until the vegetables and turkey are tender.
7. Remove the bay leaf before serving.
8. Serve hot, garnished with fresh parsley.

Nutrition Info (Per Serving):

- Calories: 240
- Protein: 26g
- Carbohydrates: 24g
- Dietary Fiber: 4g
- Sugars: 12g
- Total Fat: 6g
- Saturated Fat: 1g
- Sodium: 150mg

Serves:

- **4 servings**

Cooking Time:

- **Total: 35 minutes**

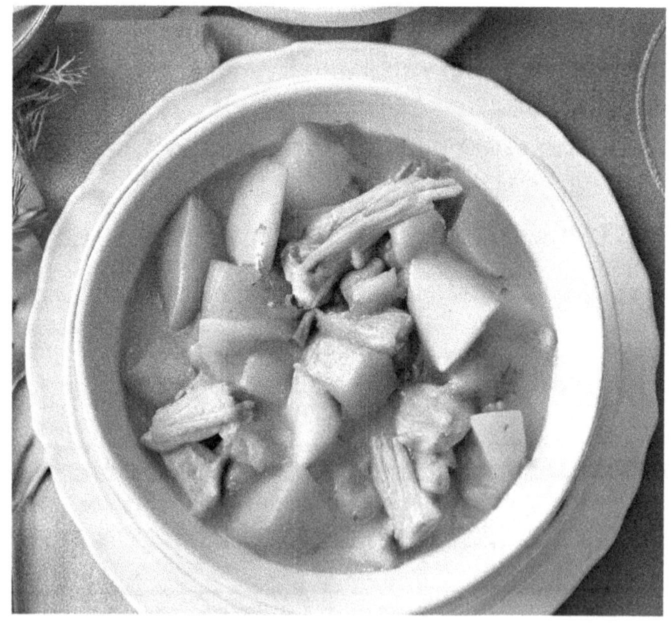

4. Chicken Rice Paper Rolls

Ingredients:

- 1 pound of cooked chicken breast, shredded
- 1 cup of julienned carrots
- 1 cup of julienned cucumber
- 1 cup of shredded lettuce
- 1/4 cup of fresh mint leaves
- 12 rice paper wrappers
- 1 tablespoon of low-sodium soy sauce
- 1 tablespoon of rice vinegar (if tolerated)
- 1 teaspoon of honey
- 1 teaspoon of sesame oil (optional)

Instructions:

1. Prepare a large bowl of warm water. Dip one rice paper wrapper into the warm water for about 10-15 seconds until it softens.
2. Place the softened wrapper on a clean, damp kitchen towel.
3. In the center of the wrapper, place a small amount of shredded chicken, julienned carrots, cucumber, shredded lettuce, and mint leaves.
4. Fold the bottom of the wrapper over the filling, then fold in the sides and roll tightly.
5. Repeat with the remaining wrappers and filling.
6. In a small bowl, mix the low-sodium soy sauce, rice vinegar (if tolerated), honey, and sesame oil (if using) to make a dipping sauce.
7. Serve the rolls with the dipping sauce.

Nutrition Info (Per Serving):

- Calories: 120
- Protein: 15g
- Carbohydrates: 12g
- Dietary Fiber: 2g
- Sugars: 3g
- Total Fat: 3g
- Saturated Fat: 0.5g
- Sodium: 100mg

Serves:

- **12 rolls**

Cooking Time:

- **Total: 20 minutes**

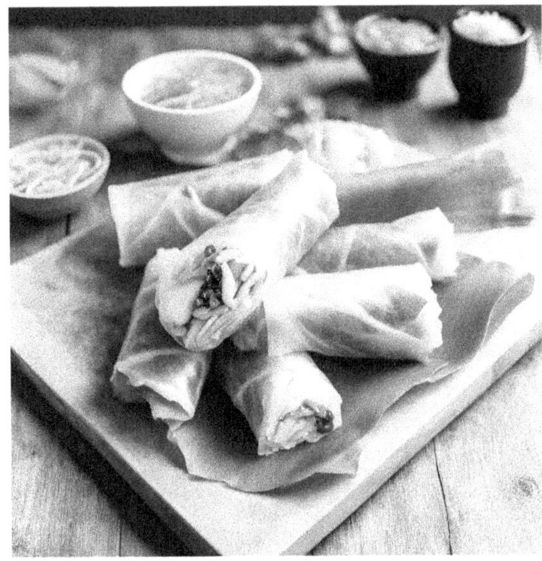

5. Poached Turkey in Ginger Broth

Ingredients:

- 1 pound turkey breast, cut into strips
- 4 cups low-sodium chicken broth
- 1-inch piece fresh ginger, peeled and sliced
- 2 medium carrots, sliced
- 2 celery stalks, sliced
- Fresh parsley for garnish

Instructions:

1. In a large pot, bring the chicken broth to a simmer.
2. Add the ginger, carrots, and celery, and simmer for 10 minutes until the vegetables are tender.
3. Add the turkey breast strips and poach for 10-12 minutes until the turkey is cooked through.
4. Remove the ginger slices before serving.
5. Serve hot, garnished with fresh parsley.

Nutrition Info (Per Serving):

- Calories: 180
- Protein: 30g
- Carbohydrates: 6g
- Dietary Fiber: 2g
- Sugars: 3g
- Total Fat: 3g
- Saturated Fat: 1g
- Sodium: 120mg

Serves:

- **4 servings**

Cooking Time:

- **Total: 25 minutes**

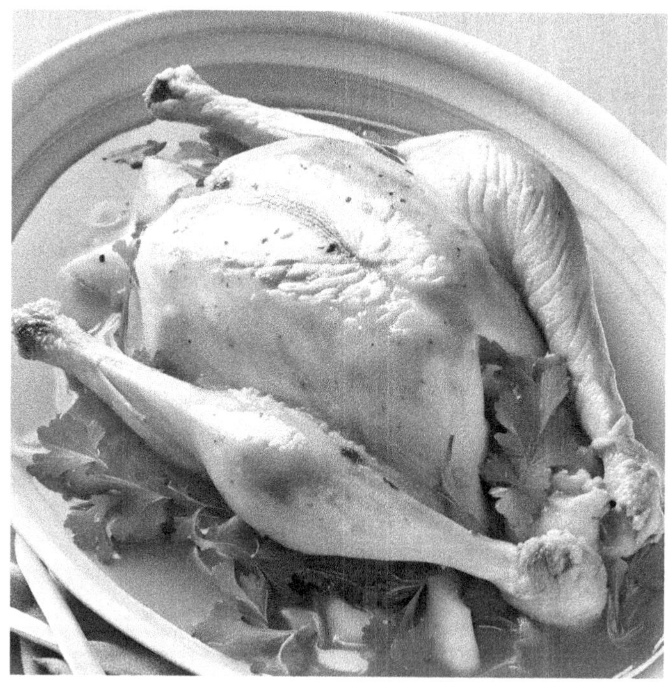

6. Turkey Casserole with Broccoli

Ingredients:

- 1 pound ground turkey
- 4 cups broccoli florets
- 2 cups cooked brown rice
- 1 cup unsweetened almond milk
- 1/2 cup grated low-fat cheese (optional)
- 1 teaspoon dried thyme
- 1 tablespoon olive oil

Instructions:

1. Preheat the oven to 375°F (190°C).
2. In a large skillet, heat the olive oil over medium heat. Add the ground turkey and cook until browned.
3. Steam the broccoli florets until tender, about 5 minutes.
4. In a large bowl, combine the cooked turkey, broccoli, cooked brown rice, almond milk, dried thyme, and grated cheese (if using).
5. Transfer the mixture to a greased casserole dish.
6. Bake for 25-30 minutes until heated through and the top is slightly golden.
7. Serve hot.

Nutrition Info (Per Serving):

- Calories: 280
- Protein: 25g
- Carbohydrates: 24g
- Dietary Fiber: 5g
- Sugars: 3g
- Total Fat: 10g
- Saturated Fat: 2g
- Sodium: 180mg

Serves:

- **6 servings**

Cooking Time:

- **Total: 40 minutes**

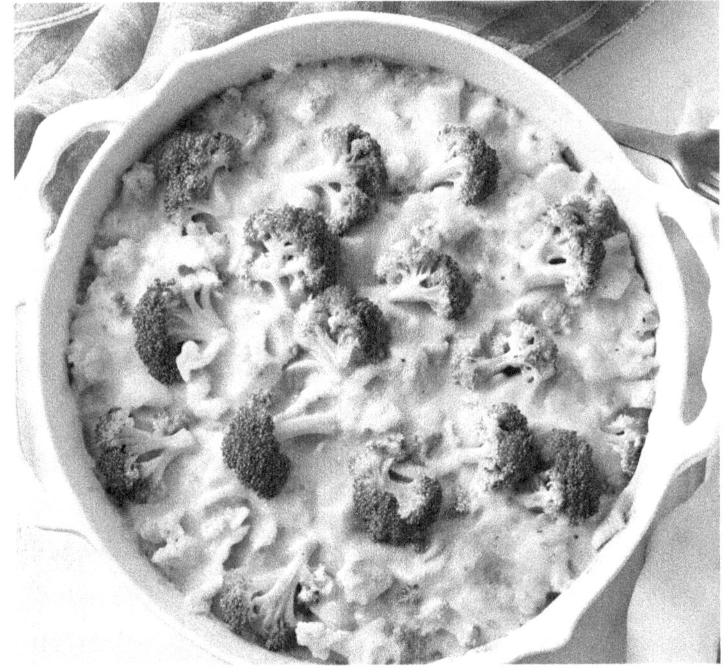

7. Chicken Gnocchi Soup

Ingredients:

- 1 pound chicken breast, cooked and shredded
- 1 cup gnocchi
- 4 cups low-sodium chicken broth
- 1 cup unsweetened almond milk
- 2 medium carrots, diced
- 2 celery stalks, diced
- 1 teaspoon dried thyme
- 1 tablespoon olive oil
- 2 cups fresh spinach, chopped

Instructions:

1. In a large pot, heat the olive oil over medium heat. Add the diced carrots and celery, and cook for 5 minutes until slightly softened.
2. Add the chicken broth and dried thyme, and bring to a boil.
3. Stir in the gnocchi and cook according to package instructions until tender.
4. Add the shredded chicken and almond milk, and simmer for an additional 5 minutes.
5. Stir in the chopped spinach and cook until wilted.
6. Serve hot.

Nutrition Info (Per Serving):

- Calories: 250
- Protein: 25g
- Carbohydrates: 20g
- Dietary Fiber: 4g
- Sugars: 3g
- Total Fat: 7g
- Saturated Fat: 1g
- Sodium: 150mg

Serves:

- **6 servings**

Cooking Time:

- **Total: 30 minutes**

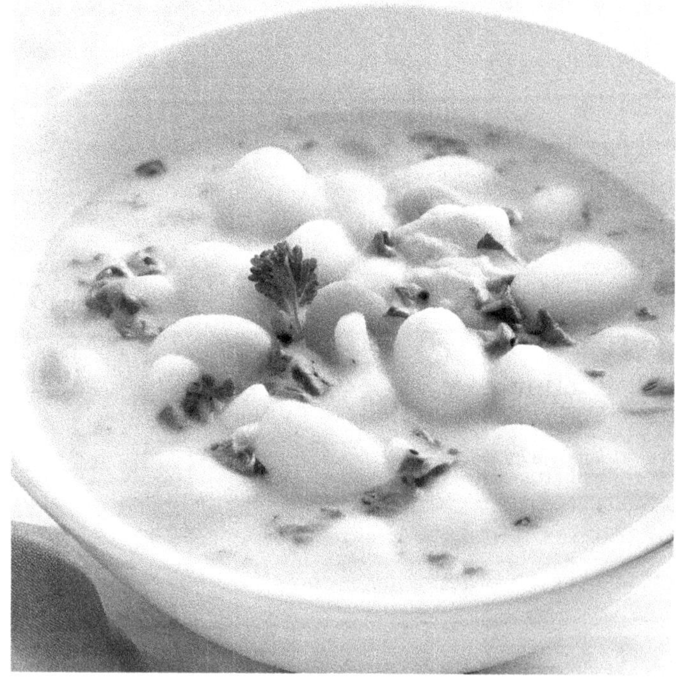

8. Turkey and Zucchini Patties

Ingredients:

- 1 pound ground turkey
- 1 cup grated zucchini
- 1/4 cup whole wheat breadcrumbs
- 1 large egg
- 1 teaspoon dried oregano
- 1 tablespoon olive oil
- Fresh parsley for garnish

Instructions:

1. In a large bowl, combine the ground turkey, grated zucchini, breadcrumbs, egg, and dried oregano. Mix well.
2. Form the mixture into 8 patties.
3. Heat the olive oil in a large skillet over medium heat.
4. Cook the patties for 5-6 minutes on each side until golden brown and cooked through.
5. Serve hot, garnished with fresh parsley.

Nutrition Info (Per Serving):

- Calories: 180
- Protein: 22g
- Carbohydrates: 5g
- Dietary Fiber: 1g
- Sugars: 1g
- Total Fat: 8g
- Saturated Fat: 2g
- Sodium: 100mg

Serves:

- **4 servings (2 patties per serving)**

Cooking Time:

- **Total: 20 minutes**

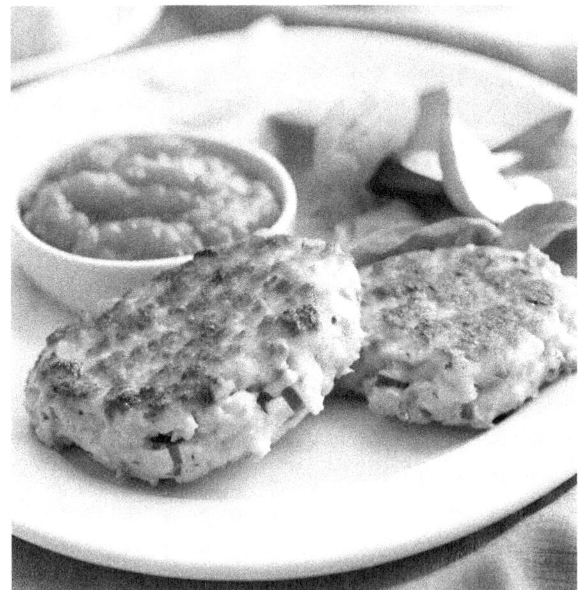

9. Turkey Spinach Quiche

Ingredients:

- 1 premade whole wheat pie crust
- 1 cup cooked ground turkey
- 2 cups fresh spinach, chopped
- 4 large eggs
- 1 cup unsweetened almond milk
- 1/2 cup grated low-fat cheese (optional)
- 1 teaspoon dried basil

Instructions:

1. Preheat the oven to 375°F (190°C).
2. Place the pie crust in a pie dish and set aside.
3. In a large bowl, whisk together the eggs, almond milk, and dried basil.
4. Spread the cooked ground turkey and chopped spinach evenly in the pie crust.
5. Pour the egg mixture over the turkey and spinach.
6. Sprinkle with grated cheese (if using).
7. Bake for 35-40 minutes until the quiche is set and lightly golden.
8. Let cool slightly before slicing and serving.

Nutrition Info (Per Serving):

- Calories: 220
- Protein: 18g
- Carbohydrates: 15g
- Dietary Fiber: 2g
- Sugars: 1g
- Total Fat: 11g
- Saturated Fat: 3g
- Sodium: 180mg

Serves:

- **6 servings**

Cooking Time:

- **Total: 45 minutes**

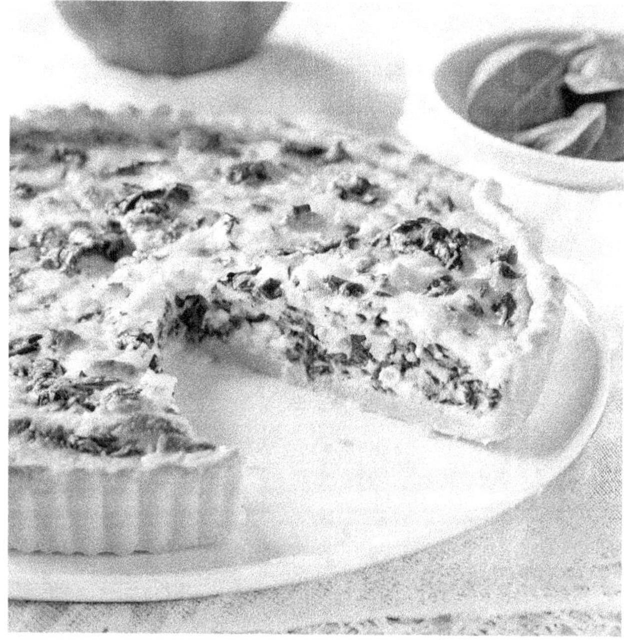

10. Chicken and Pear Salad

Ingredients:

- 2 cups cooked chicken breast, shredded
- 2 ripe pears, sliced
- 4 cups mixed greens
- 1/4 cup walnuts, chopped
- 1/4 cup feta cheese, crumbled (optional)
- 2 tablespoons olive oil
- 1 tablespoon honey
- 1 tablespoon lemon juice (if tolerated)

Instructions:

1. In a large salad bowl, combine the mixed greens, shredded chicken, sliced pears, walnuts, and feta cheese (if using).
2. In a small bowl, whisk together the olive oil, honey, and lemon juice (if tolerated).
3. Drizzle the dressing over the salad and toss gently to combine.
4. Serve immediately.

Nutrition Info (Per Serving):

- Calories: 250
- Protein: 20g
- Carbohydrates: 18g
- Dietary Fiber: 4g
- Sugars: 12g
- Total Fat: 12g
- Saturated Fat: 3g
- Sodium: 120mg

Serves:

- **4 servings**

Cooking Time:

- **Total: 10 minutes**

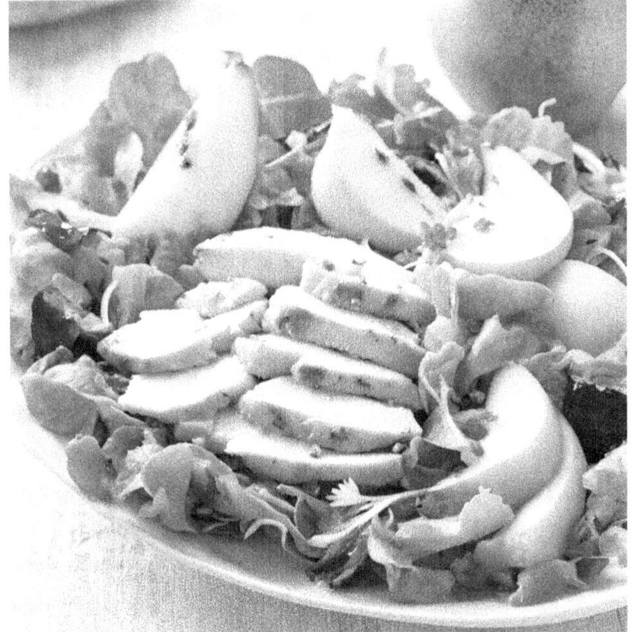

11. Roast Turkey with Squash

Ingredients:

- 1 turkey breast (about 2 pounds)
- 2 tablespoons of olive oil
- 1 teaspoon of dried thyme
- 1 teaspoon of dried rosemary
- 2 medium butternut squash, peeled, seeded, and cut into cubes
- Fresh parsley for garnish

Instructions:

1. Preheat the oven to 375°F (190°C).
2. Rub the turkey breast with 1 tablespoon of olive oil and sprinkle with dried thyme and rosemary.
3. Place the turkey breast in a roasting pan.
4. Toss the butternut squash cubes with the remaining olive oil and spread them around the turkey in the roasting pan.
5. Roast for 45-50 minutes, or until the turkey is cooked through and the internal temperature reaches 165°F (75°C).
6. Let the turkey rest for 10 minutes before slicing.
7. Serve the turkey with roasted squash, garnished with fresh parsley.

Nutrition Info (Per Serving):

- Calories: 300
- Protein: 30g
- Carbohydrates: 20g
- Dietary Fiber: 4g
- Sugars: 5g
- Total Fat: 12g
- Saturated Fat: 2g
- Sodium: 100mg

Serves:

- **4 servings**

Cooking Time:

- **Total: 60 minutes**

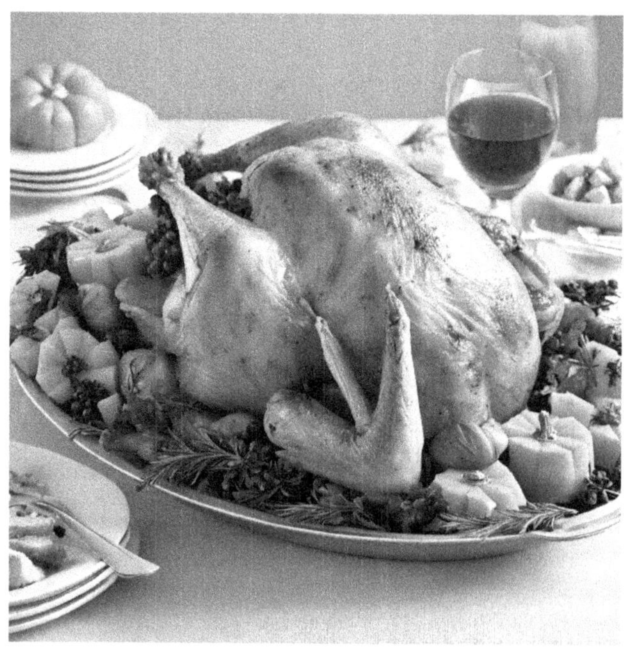

12. Turkey Pilaf

Ingredients:

- 1 pound ground turkey
- 1 cup brown rice
- 2 medium carrots, diced
- 2 celery stalks, diced
- 4 cups low-sodium chicken broth
- 1 tablespoon olive oil
- 1 teaspoon dried thyme
- 1 teaspoon dried oregano
- Fresh parsley for garnish

Instructions:

1. In a large pot, heat the olive oil over medium heat.
2. Add the ground turkey and cook until browned.
3. Add the diced carrots and celery, and cook for 5 minutes until slightly softened.
4. Stir in the brown rice, dried thyme, and oregano.
5. Pour in the chicken broth and bring to a boil.
6. Reduce heat to low, cover, and simmer for 30-35 minutes, or until the rice is tender and the liquid is absorbed.
7. Serve hot, garnished with fresh parsley.

Nutrition Info (Per Serving):

- Calories: 280
- Protein: 25g
- Carbohydrates: 30g
- Dietary Fiber: 4g
- Sugars: 4g
- Total Fat: 8g
- Saturated Fat: 2g
- Sodium: 180mg

Serves:

- **4 servings**

Cooking Time:

- **Total: 40 minutes**

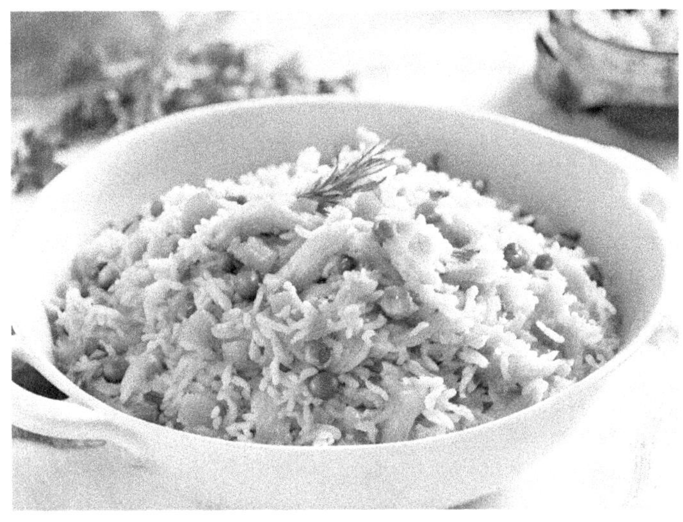

13. Chicken Pea Soup

Ingredients:

- 1 pound chicken breast, cooked and shredded
- 4 cups low-sodium chicken broth
- 2 cups frozen peas
- 2 medium carrots, diced
- 2 celery stalks, diced
- 1 tablespoon olive oil
- 1 teaspoon dried thyme
- Fresh parsley for garnish

Instructions:

1. In a large pot, heat the olive oil over medium heat.
2. Add the diced carrots and celery, and cook for 5 minutes until slightly softened.
3. Add the chicken broth and dried thyme, and bring to a boil.
4. Stir in the frozen peas and shredded chicken, and cook for an additional 5 minutes until the peas are tender and the soup is heated through.
5. Serve hot, garnished with fresh parsley.

Nutrition Info (Per Serving):

- Calories: 220
- Protein: 25g
- Carbohydrates: 15g
- Dietary Fiber: 5g
- Sugars: 6g
- Total Fat: 6g
- Saturated Fat: 1g
- Sodium: 150mg

Serves:

- **4 servings**

Cooking Time:

- **Total: 20 minutes**

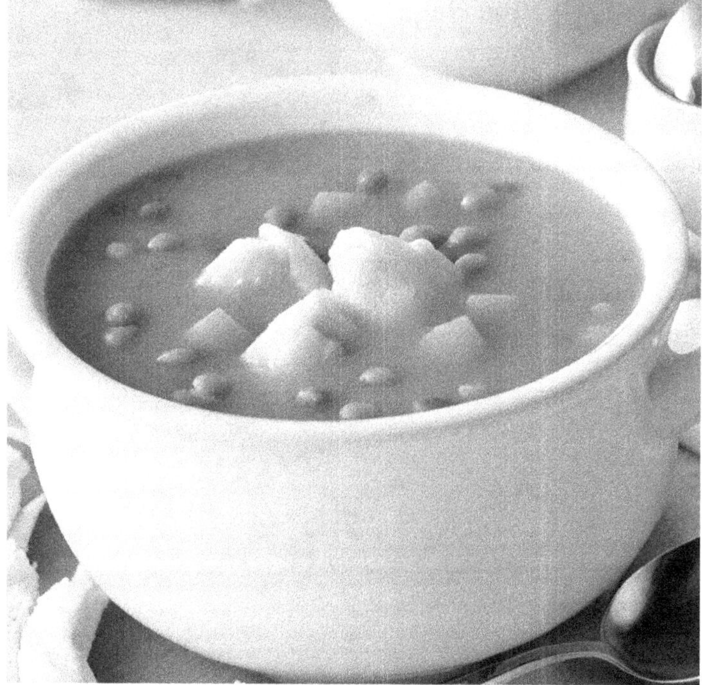

14. Turkey and Vegetable Loaf

Ingredients:

- 1 pound ground turkey
- 1 cup grated zucchini
- 1 cup grated carrot
- 1/2 cup whole wheat breadcrumbs
- 1 large egg
- 1 teaspoon dried thyme
- 1 teaspoon dried basil
- 1 tablespoon olive oil

Instructions:

1. Preheat the oven to 375°F (190°C).
2. In a large bowl, combine the ground turkey, grated zucchini, grated carrot, breadcrumbs, egg, dried thyme, and dried basil. Mix well.
3. Transfer the mixture to a greased loaf pan and smooth the top.
4. Bake for 45-50 minutes, or until the loaf is cooked through and the internal temperature reaches 165°F (75°C).
5. Let the loaf rest for 10 minutes before slicing and serving.

Nutrition Info (Per Serving):

- Calories: 180
- Protein: 22g
- Carbohydrates: 10g
- Dietary Fiber: 2g
- Sugars: 3g
- Total Fat: 6g
- Saturated Fat: 1g
- Sodium: 100mg

Serves:

- **4 servings**

Cooking Time:

- **Total: 60 minutes**

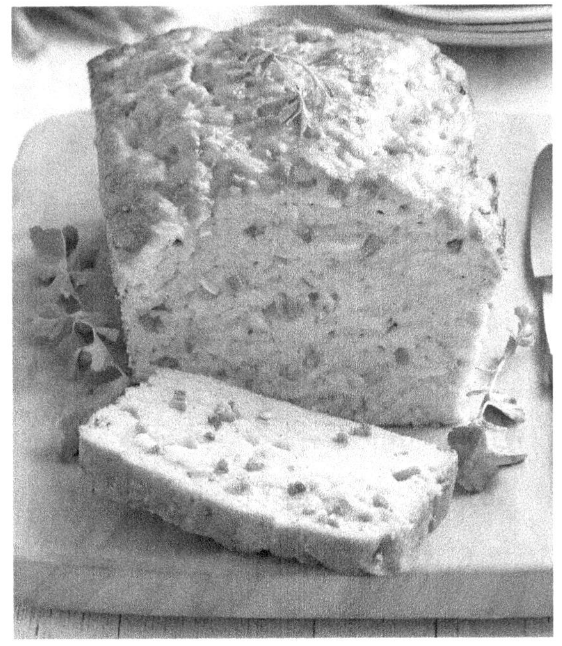

15. Roast Chicken with Herbs

Ingredients:

- 1 whole chicken (about 4 pounds)
- 2 tablespoons of olive oil
- 1 teaspoon of dried thyme
- 1 teaspoon of dried rosemary
- 1 teaspoon of dried oregano
- 1 lemon, halved (if tolerated)
- Fresh parsley for garnish

Instructions:

1. Preheat the oven to 375°F (190°C).
2. Rub the chicken with olive oil and sprinkle with dried thyme, rosemary, and oregano.
3. Place the lemon halves (if tolerated) inside the cavity of the chicken.
4. Place the chicken on a roasting rack in a roasting pan.
5. Roast for 1 hour and 20 minutes, or until the internal temperature reaches 165°F (75°C).
6. Let the chicken rest for 10 minutes before carving.
7. Serve garnished with fresh parsley.

Nutrition Info (Per Serving):

- Calories: 350
- Protein: 40g
- Carbohydrates: 2g
- Dietary Fiber: 1g
- Sugars: 0g
- Total Fat: 20g
- Saturated Fat: 5g
- Sodium: 100mg

Serves:

- **6 servings**

Cooking Time:

- **Total: 1 hour and 30 minutes**

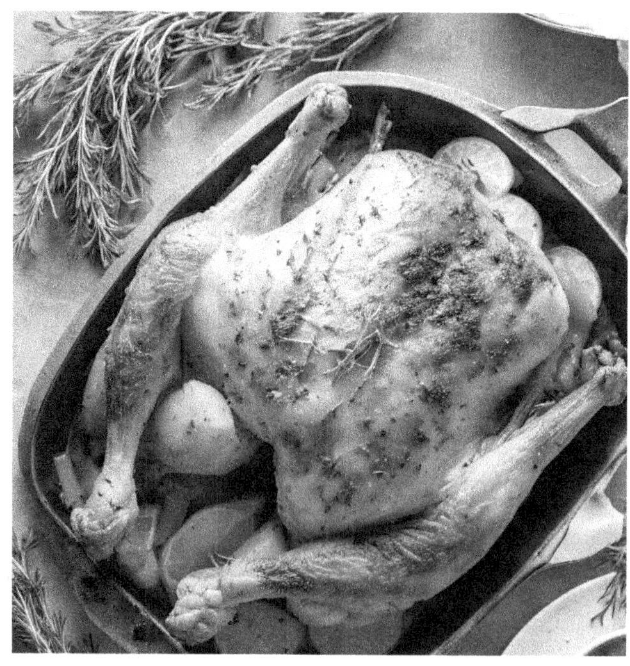

16. Chicken Tenderloins in Broth

Ingredients:

- 1 pound chicken tenderloins
- 4 cups low-sodium chicken broth
- 2 medium carrots, sliced
- 2 celery stalks, sliced
- 1 tablespoon olive oil
- 1 teaspoon dried thyme
- Fresh parsley for garnish

Instructions:

1. In a large pot, heat the olive oil over medium heat.
2. Add the chicken tenderloins and cook until lightly browned.
3. Add the sliced carrots and celery, and cook for 5 minutes until slightly softened.
4. Pour in the chicken broth and add the dried thyme. Bring to a boil.
5. Reduce heat to low and simmer for 15 minutes until the chicken is cooked through and the vegetables are tender.
6. Serve hot, garnished with fresh parsley.

Nutrition Info (Per Serving):

- Calories: 180
- Protein: 28g
- Carbohydrates: 5g
- Dietary Fiber: 2g
- Sugars: 3g
- Total Fat: 5g
- Saturated Fat: 1g
- Sodium: 120mg

Serves:

- **4 servings**

Cooking Time:

- **Total: 25 minutes**

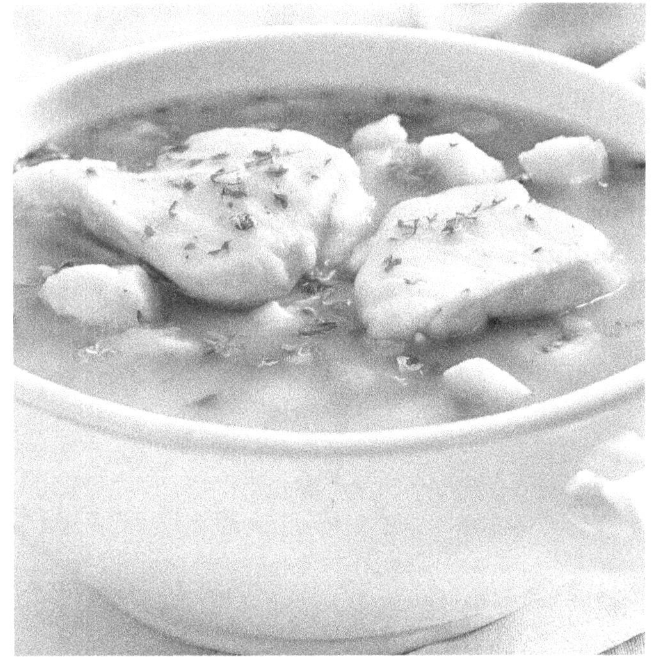

17. Grilled Turkey Breast

Ingredients:

- 1 pound turkey breast fillets
- 2 tablespoons of olive oil
- 1 teaspoon of dried thyme
- 1 teaspoon of dried rosemary
- Fresh lemon wedges (if tolerated) for serving

Instructions:

1. Preheat the grill to medium-high heat.
2. Brush the turkey breast fillets with olive oil and sprinkle with dried thyme and rosemary.
3. Grill the turkey breast fillets for 5-6 minutes on each side, or until the internal temperature reaches 165°F (75°C).
4. Serve with fresh lemon wedges (if tolerated).

Nutrition Info (Per Serving):

- Calories: 210
- Protein: 35g
- Carbohydrates: 1g
- Dietary Fiber: 0g
- Sugars: 0g
- Total Fat: 8g
- Saturated Fat: 1g
- Sodium: 80mg

Serves:

- **4 servings**

Cooking Time:

- **Total: 15 minutes**

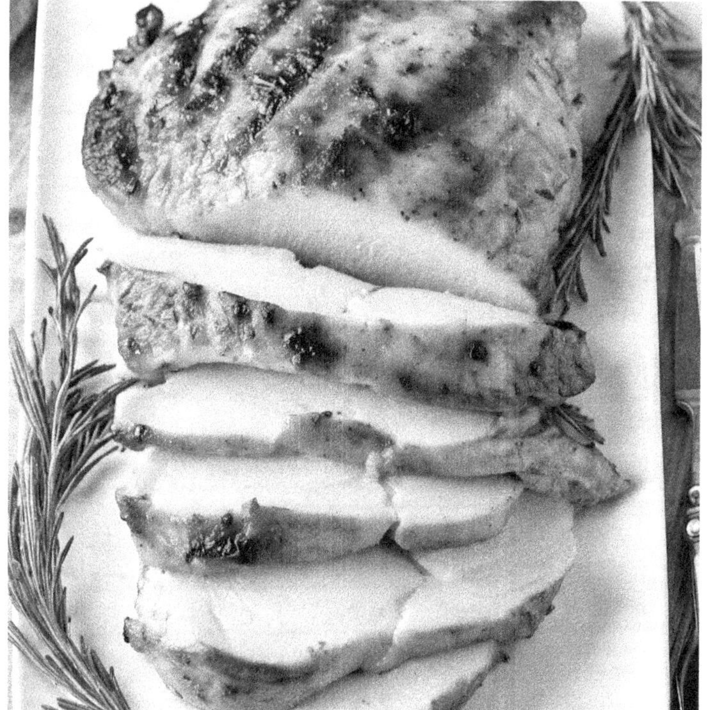

18. Chicken Porridge

Ingredients:

- 1 cup jasmine rice
- 8 cups low-sodium chicken broth
- 1 pound chicken breast, cooked and shredded
- 2 medium carrots, diced
- 2 celery stalks, diced
- 1 tablespoon fresh ginger, grated
- Fresh cilantro for garnish

Instructions:

1. Rinse the jasmine rice under cold water until the water runs clear.
2. In a large pot, bring the chicken broth to a boil.
3. Add the rice to the pot and reduce heat to low. Simmer for about 1 hour, stirring occasionally, until the rice has broken down and the porridge has thickened.
4. Add the shredded chicken, diced carrots, celery, and grated ginger. Simmer for an additional 10 minutes until the vegetables are tender.
5. Serve hot, garnished with fresh cilantro.

Nutrition Info (Per Serving):

- Calories: 250
- Protein: 20g
- Carbohydrates: 32g
- Dietary Fiber: 2g
- Sugars: 2g
- Total Fat: 5g
- Saturated Fat: 1g
- Sodium: 150mg

Serves:

- **6 servings**

Cooking Time:

- **Total: 70 minutes**

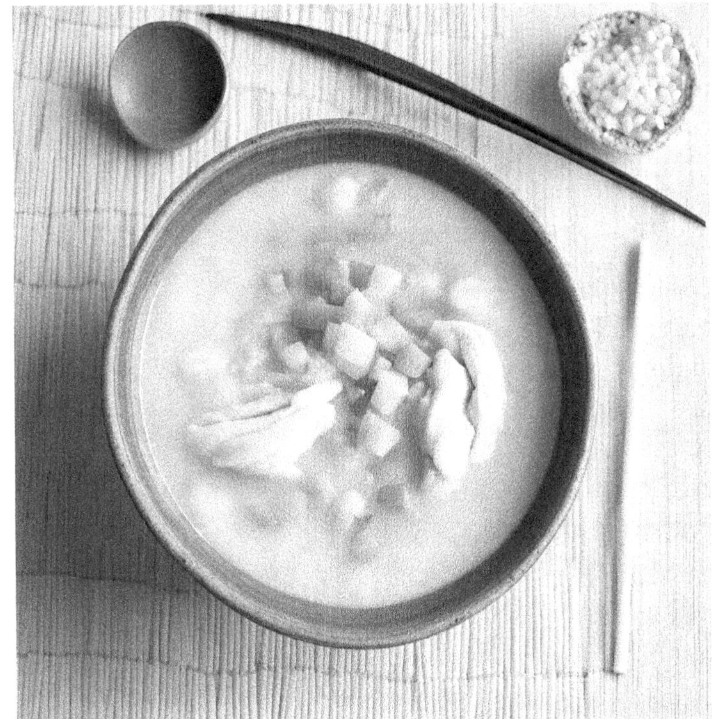

19. Chicken with Mashed Potatoes

Ingredients:

- 4 boneless, skinless chicken breasts
- 2 tablespoons olive oil
- 1 teaspoon dried thyme
- 1 teaspoon dried rosemary
- 2 pounds potatoes, peeled and cubed
- 1/2 cup unsweetened almond milk
- 2 tablespoons unsalted butter
- Fresh parsley for garnish

Instructions:

1. Preheat the oven to 375°F (190°C).
2. Rub the chicken breasts with olive oil and sprinkle with dried thyme and rosemary.
3. Place the chicken breasts in a baking dish and bake for 25-30 minutes, or until the internal temperature reaches 165°F (75°C).
4. Meanwhile, in a large pot, boil the cubed potatoes until tender, about 15 minutes.
5. Drain the potatoes and return them to the pot. Add the almond milk and unsalted butter, and mash until smooth.
6. Serve the baked chicken with mashed potatoes, garnished with fresh parsley.

Nutrition Info (Per Serving):

- Calories: 320
- Protein: 28g
- Carbohydrates: 35g
- Dietary Fiber: 5g
- Sugars: 2g
- Total Fat: 9g
- Saturated Fat: 3g
- Sodium: 150mg

Serves:

- **4 servings**

Cooking Time:

- **Total: 40 minutes**

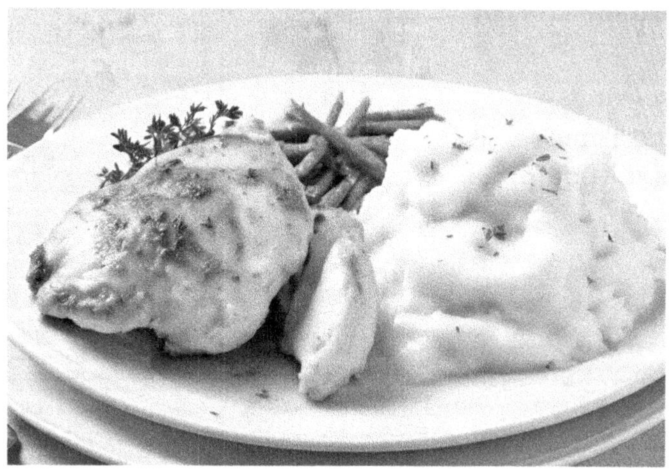

20. Baked Turkey Meatloaf

Ingredients:

- 1 pound ground turkey
- 1/2 cup whole wheat breadcrumbs
- 1/4 cup unsweetened almond milk
- 1 large egg
- 1 cup grated zucchini
- 1 teaspoon dried basil
- 1 teaspoon dried oregano
- 1 tablespoon olive oil

Instructions:

1. Preheat the oven to 375°F (190°C).
2. In a large bowl, combine the ground turkey, breadcrumbs, almond milk, egg, grated zucchini, dried basil, and dried oregano. Mix well.
3. Transfer the mixture to a greased loaf pan and smooth the top.
4. Bake for 45-50 minutes, or until the internal temperature reaches 165°F (75°C).
5. Let the meatloaf rest for 10 minutes before slicing and serving.

Nutrition Info (Per Serving):

- Calories: 200
- Protein: 22g
- Carbohydrates: 10g
- Dietary Fiber: 2g
- Sugars: 1g
- Total Fat: 9g
- Saturated Fat: 2g
- Sodium: 120mg

Serves:

- **4 servings**

Cooking Time:

- **Total: 60 minutes**

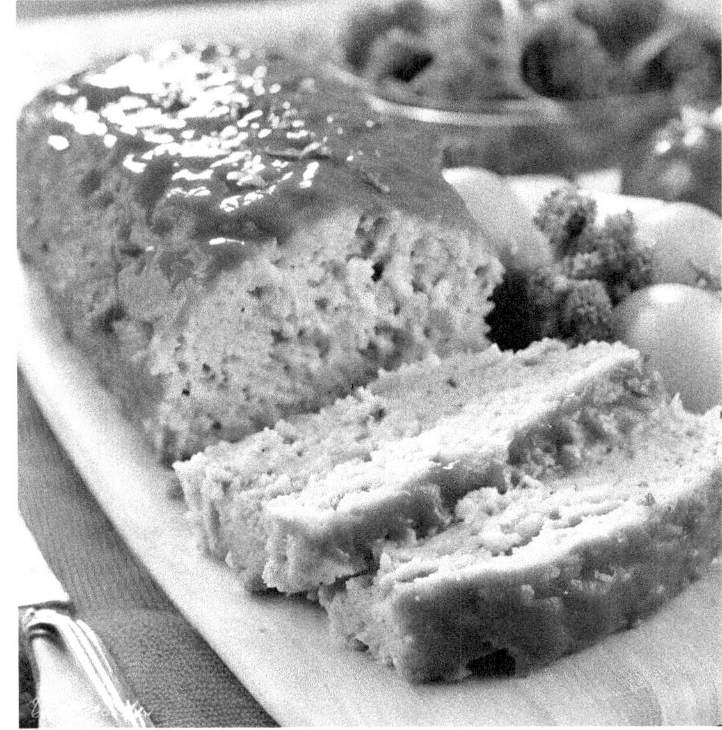

21. Turkey Apple Burgers

Ingredients:

- 1 pound ground turkey
- 1 apple, grated
- 1/4 cup whole wheat breadcrumbs
- 1 large egg
- 1 teaspoon dried thyme
- 1 tablespoon olive oil

Instructions:

1. In a large bowl, combine the ground turkey, grated apple, breadcrumbs, egg, and dried thyme. Mix well.
2. Form the mixture into 4 patties.
3. Heat the olive oil in a large skillet over medium heat.
4. Cook the patties for 5-6 minutes on each side, until golden brown and cooked through.
5. Serve on whole grain buns or on a bed of lettuce, as preferred.

Nutrition Info (Per Serving):

- Calories: 210
- Protein: 22g
- Carbohydrates: 12g
- Dietary Fiber: 2g
- Sugars: 4g
- Total Fat: 8g
- Saturated Fat: 2g
- Sodium: 100mg

Serves:

- **4 servings**

Cooking Time:

- **Total: 20 minutes**

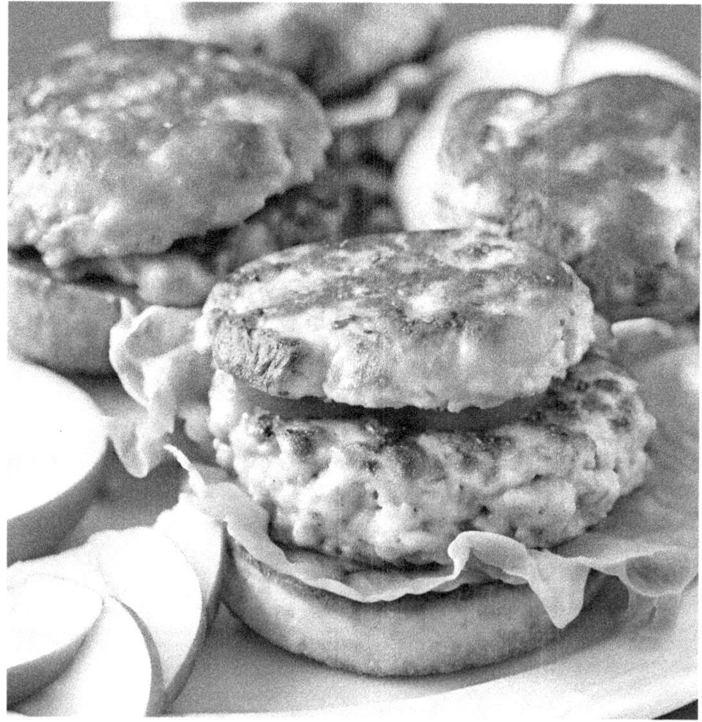

22. Chicken and Vegetable Skewers

Ingredients:

- 1 pound boneless, skinless chicken breast, cut into cubes
- 2 medium zucchini, sliced
- 1 cup mushrooms, halved
- 1 cup cherry tomatoes (if tolerated)
- 1/4 cup olive oil
- 1 teaspoon dried rosemary
- 1 teaspoon dried thyme
- Fresh parsley for garnish

Instructions:

1. Preheat the grill to medium-high heat.
2. In a large bowl, combine the olive oil, dried rosemary, and dried thyme.
3. Add the chicken cubes, zucchini, mushrooms, and cherry tomatoes (if tolerated) to the bowl, and toss to coat.
4. Thread the chicken and vegetables onto skewers.
5. Grill the skewers for 10-12 minutes, turning occasionally, until the chicken is cooked through and the vegetables are tender.
6. Serve hot, garnished with fresh parsley.

Nutrition Info (Per Serving):

- Calories: 250
- Protein: 25g
- Carbohydrates: 10g
- Dietary Fiber: 3g
- Sugars: 5g
- Total Fat: 12g
- Saturated Fat: 2g
- Sodium: 120mg

Serves:

- **4 servings**

Cooking Time:

- **Total: 20 minutes**

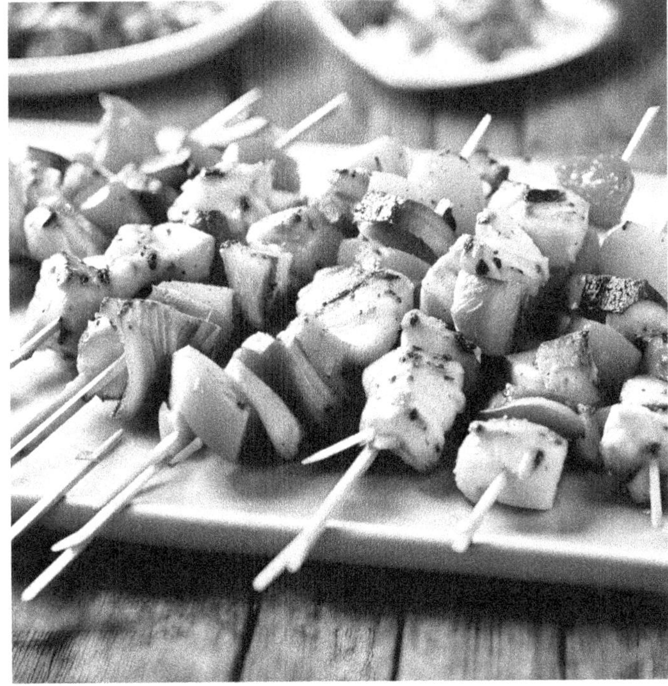

23. Slow Cooker Chicken with Carrots

Ingredients:

- 4 boneless, skinless chicken breasts
- 4 large carrots, sliced
- 2 celery stalks, sliced
- 4 cups low-sodium chicken broth
- 1 teaspoon dried thyme
- 1 teaspoon dried rosemary
- 1 tablespoon olive oil
- Fresh parsley for garnish

Instructions:

1. Heat the olive oil in a skillet over medium heat. Sear the chicken breasts for 2-3 minutes on each side until lightly browned.
2. Place the seared chicken breasts, carrots, and celery in the slow cooker.
3. Pour the chicken broth over the ingredients.
4. Sprinkle with dried thyme and rosemary.
5. Cover and cook on low for 6-8 hours or on high for 3-4 hours until the chicken is cooked through and the vegetables are tender.
6. Serve hot, garnished with fresh parsley.

Nutrition Info (Per Serving):

- Calories: 250
- Protein: 30g
- Carbohydrates: 10g
- Dietary Fiber: 3g
- Sugars: 5g
- Total Fat: 8g
- Saturated Fat: 1g
- Sodium: 150mg

Serves:

- **4 servings**

Cooking Time:

- **Total: 6-8 hours (slow cooker)**

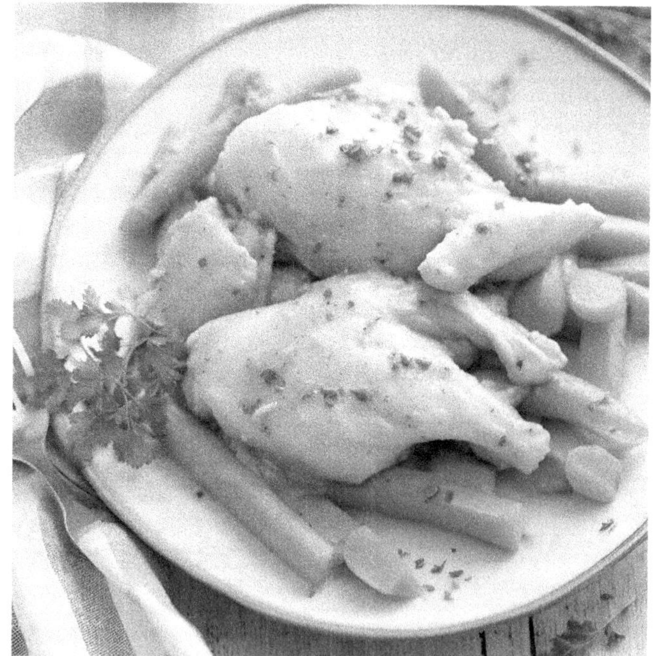

24. Stuffed Chicken Breast

Ingredients:

- 4 boneless, skinless chicken breasts
- 1 cup fresh spinach, chopped
- 1/2 cup low-fat feta cheese, crumbled
- 1/4 cup sun-dried tomatoes (if tolerated), chopped
- 1 tablespoon olive oil
- 1 teaspoon dried oregano

Instructions:

1. Preheat the oven to 375°F (190°C).
2. Cut a pocket into each chicken breast by slicing horizontally, but not all the way through.
3. In a bowl, mix the chopped spinach, feta cheese, and sun-dried tomatoes (if tolerated).
4. Stuff each chicken breast with the spinach mixture and secure with toothpicks if needed.
5. Rub the chicken breasts with olive oil and sprinkle with dried oregano.
6. Place the chicken breasts in a baking dish and bake for 25-30 minutes, or until the internal temperature reaches 165°F (75°C).
7. Remove toothpicks before serving.

Nutrition Info (Per Serving):

- Calories: 280
- Protein: 35g
- Carbohydrates: 3g
- Dietary Fiber: 1g
- Sugars: 1g
- Total Fat: 14g
- Saturated Fat: 4g
- Sodium: 200mg

Serves:

- **4 servings**

Cooking Time:

- **Total: 35 minutes**

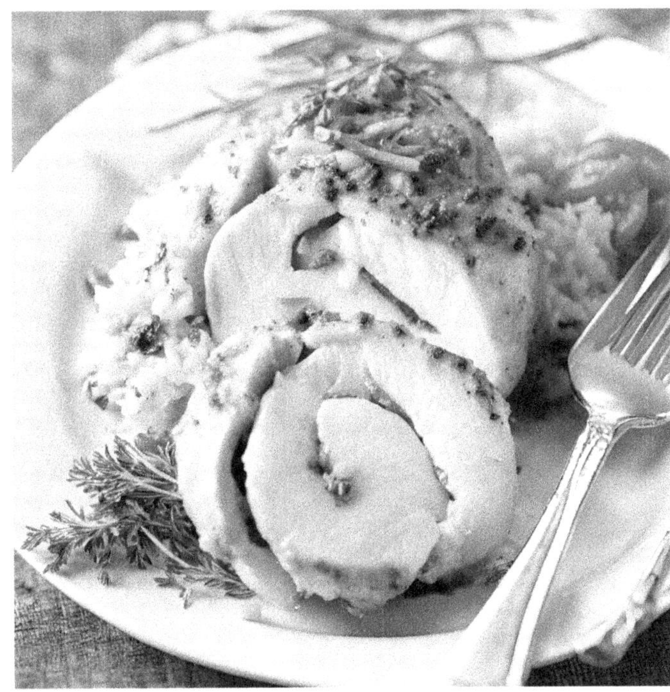

25. Turkey Quinoa Pilaf

Ingredients:

- 1 pound ground turkey
- 1 cup quinoa
- 2 cups low-sodium chicken broth
- 2 medium carrots, diced
- 2 celery stalks, diced
- 1 tablespoon olive oil
- 1 teaspoon dried thyme
- Fresh parsley for garnish

Instructions:

1. Rinse the quinoa under cold water.
2. In a large pot, heat the olive oil over medium heat. Add the ground turkey and cook until browned.
3. Add the diced carrots and celery, and cook for 5 minutes until slightly softened.
4. Stir in the quinoa and dried thyme.
5. Pour in the chicken broth and bring to a boil.
6. Reduce heat to low, cover, and simmer for 15-20 minutes, or until the quinoa is tender and the liquid is absorbed.
7. Serve hot, garnished with fresh parsley.

Nutrition Info (Per Serving):

- Calories: 280
- Protein: 25g
- Carbohydrates: 25g
- Dietary Fiber: 4g
- Sugars: 3g
- Total Fat: 9g
- Saturated Fat: 2g
- Sodium: 150mg

Serves:

- **4 servings**

Cooking Time:

- **Total: 30 minutes**

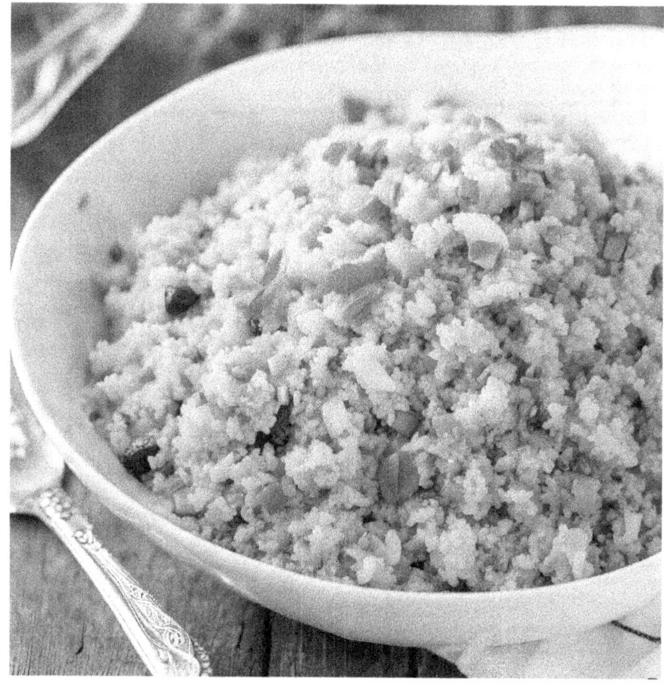

26. Turkey and Sweet Potato Stew

Ingredients:

- 1 pound turkey breast, cubed
- 2 large sweet potatoes, peeled and cubed
- 4 cups low-sodium chicken broth
- 2 medium carrots, sliced
- 2 celery stalks, sliced
- 1 tablespoon olive oil
- 1 teaspoon dried sage
- Fresh parsley for garnish

Instructions:

1. In a large pot, heat the olive oil over medium heat. Add the cubed turkey and cook until browned.
2. Add the sweet potatoes, carrots, and celery to the pot, and cook for 5 minutes until slightly softened.
3. Pour in the chicken broth and add the dried sage. Bring to a boil.
4. Reduce heat to low and simmer for 20-25 minutes, or until the sweet potatoes are tender.
5. Serve hot, garnished with fresh parsley.

Nutrition Info (Per Serving):

- Calories: 300
- Protein: 28g
- Carbohydrates: 35g
- Dietary Fiber: 5g
- Sugars: 10g
- Total Fat: 7g
- Saturated Fat: 1g
- Sodium: 180mg

Serves:

- **4 servings**

Cooking Time:

- **Total: 35 minutes**

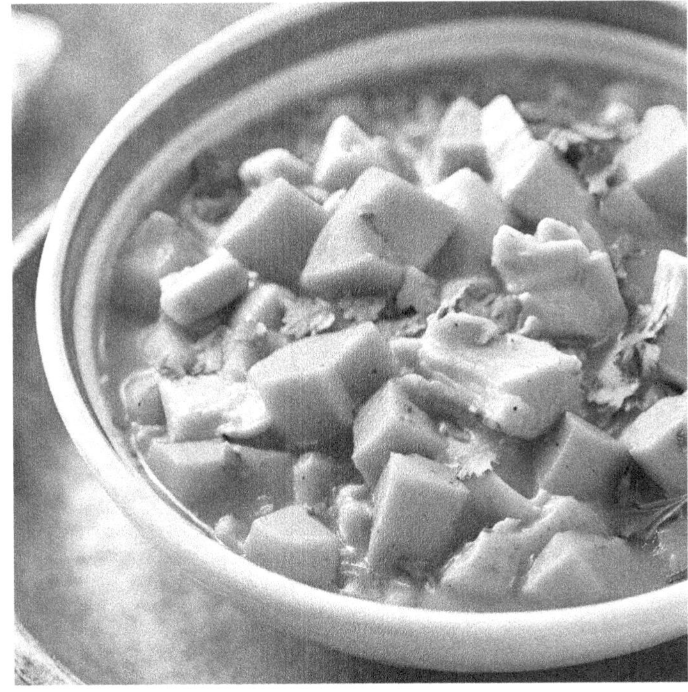

27. Oven-Roasted Turkey Breast

Ingredients:

- 1 turkey breast (about 2 pounds)
- 2 tablespoons olive oil
- 1 teaspoon dried thyme
- 1 teaspoon dried rosemary
- 1 teaspoon dried oregano
- Fresh parsley for garnish

Instructions:

1. Preheat the oven to 375°F (190°C).
2. Rub the turkey breast with olive oil and sprinkle with dried thyme, rosemary, and oregano.
3. Place the turkey breast on a roasting rack in a roasting pan.
4. Roast for 1 hour and 20 minutes, or until the internal temperature reaches 165°F (75°C).
5. Let the turkey rest for 10 minutes before slicing.
6. Serve garnished with fresh parsley.

Nutrition Info (Per Serving):

- Calories: 260
- Protein: 35g
- Carbohydrates: 1g
- Dietary Fiber: 0g
- Sugars: 0g
- Total Fat: 12g
- Saturated Fat: 3g
- Sodium: 100mg

Serves:

- **6 servings**

Cooking Time:

- **Total: 1 hour and 30 minutes**

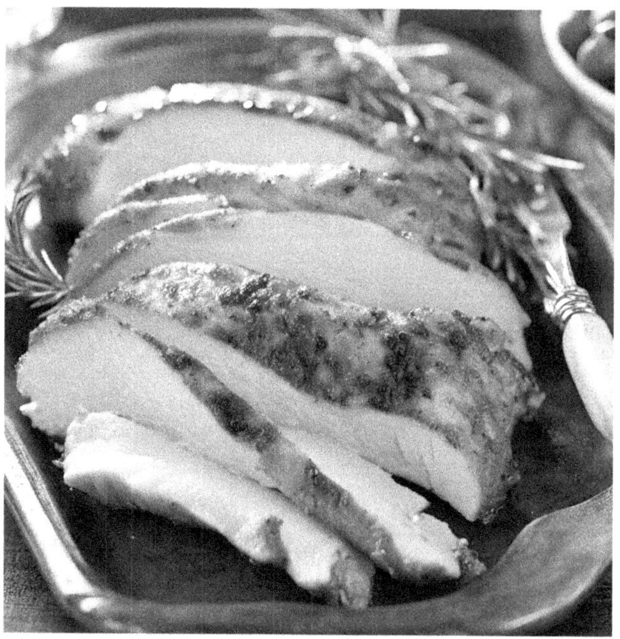

Vegetables

1. Mushroom and Barley Soup

Ingredients:

- 1 cup pearl barley
- 6 cups low-sodium vegetable broth
- 2 cups sliced mushrooms
- 2 medium carrots, diced
- 2 celery stalks, diced
- 1 tablespoon olive oil
- 1 teaspoon dried thyme
- Fresh parsley for garnish

Instructions:

1. Rinse the pearl barley under cold water.
2. In a large pot, heat the olive oil over medium heat.
3. Add the sliced mushrooms, diced carrots, and celery, and cook for 5 minutes until slightly softened.
4. Add the barley and dried thyme to the pot and stir to combine.
5. Pour in the vegetable broth and bring to a boil.
6. Reduce heat to low and simmer for 45-50 minutes, or until the barley is tender.
7. Serve hot, garnished with fresh parsley.

Nutrition Info (Per Serving):

- Calories: 200
- Protein: 5g
- Carbohydrates: 38g
- Dietary Fiber: 8g
- Sugars: 6g
- Total Fat: 4g
- Saturated Fat: 0.5g
- Sodium: 150mg

Serves:

- **6 servings**

Cooking Time:

- **Total: 60 minutes**

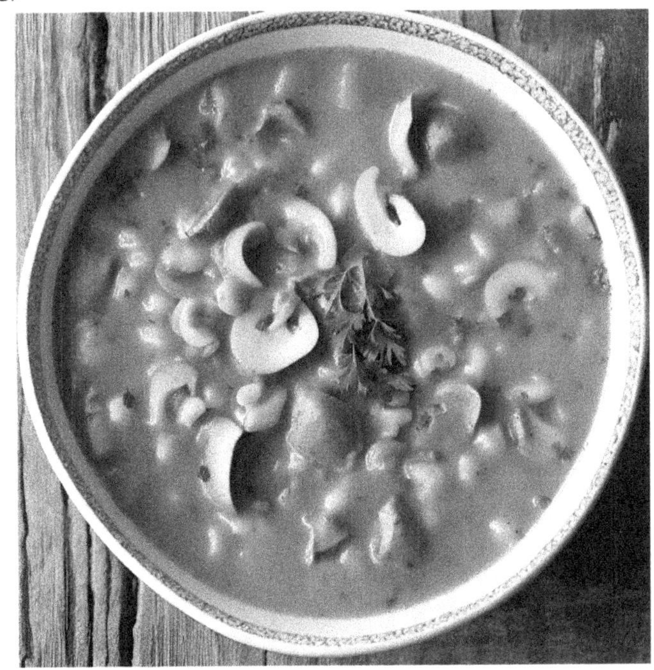

2. Grilled Eggplant with Basil

Ingredients:

- 2 medium eggplants, sliced into rounds
- 2 tablespoons olive oil
- 1/4 cup fresh basil leaves, chopped
- 1 teaspoon dried oregano
- Fresh lemon wedges (if tolerated) for serving

Instructions:

1. Preheat the grill to medium-high heat.
2. Brush the eggplant slices with olive oil and sprinkle with dried oregano.
3. Grill the eggplant slices for 3-4 minutes on each side, until tender and grill marks appear.
4. Remove from the grill and sprinkle with fresh basil.
5. Serve with fresh lemon wedges (if tolerated).

Nutrition Info (Per Serving):

- Calories: 80
- Protein: 1g
- Carbohydrates: 9g
- Dietary Fiber: 4g
- Sugars: 4g
- Total Fat: 5g
- Saturated Fat: 1g
- Sodium: 20mg

Serves:

- **4 servings**

Cooking Time:

- **Total: 15 minutes**

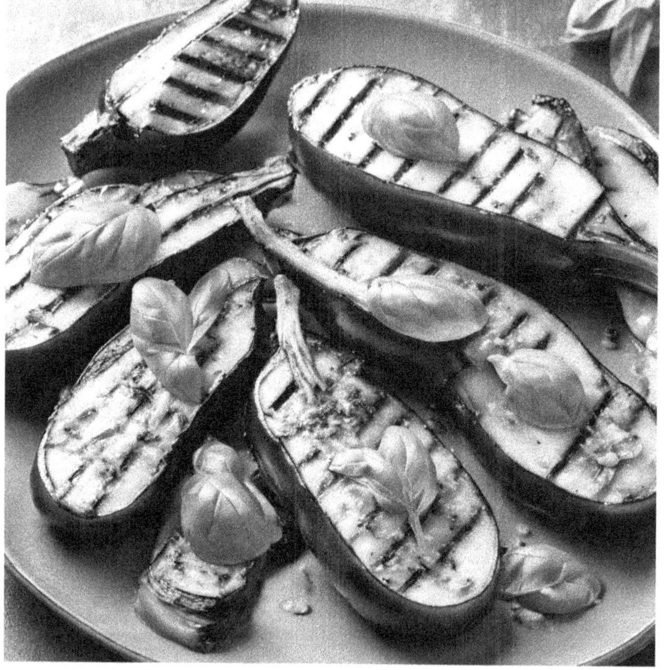

3. Squash Stew

Ingredients:

- 2 medium butternut squash, peeled and cubed
- 4 cups low-sodium vegetable broth
- 2 medium carrots, sliced
- 2 celery stalks, sliced
- 1 tablespoon olive oil
- 1 teaspoon dried thyme
- 1 teaspoon dried sage
- Fresh parsley for garnish

Instructions:

1. In a large pot, heat the olive oil over medium heat.
2. Add the cubed butternut squash, sliced carrots, and celery, and cook for 5 minutes until slightly softened.
3. Add the vegetable broth, dried thyme, and sage to the pot.
4. Bring to a boil, then reduce heat to low and simmer for 20-25 minutes, or until the vegetables are tender.
5. Serve hot, garnished with fresh parsley.

Nutrition Info (Per Serving):

- Calories: 150
- Protein: 3g
- Carbohydrates: 30g
- Dietary Fiber: 7g
- Sugars: 8g
- Total Fat: 4g
- Saturated Fat: 0.5g
- Sodium: 120mg

Serves:

- **4 servings**

Cooking Time:

- **Total: 35 minutes**

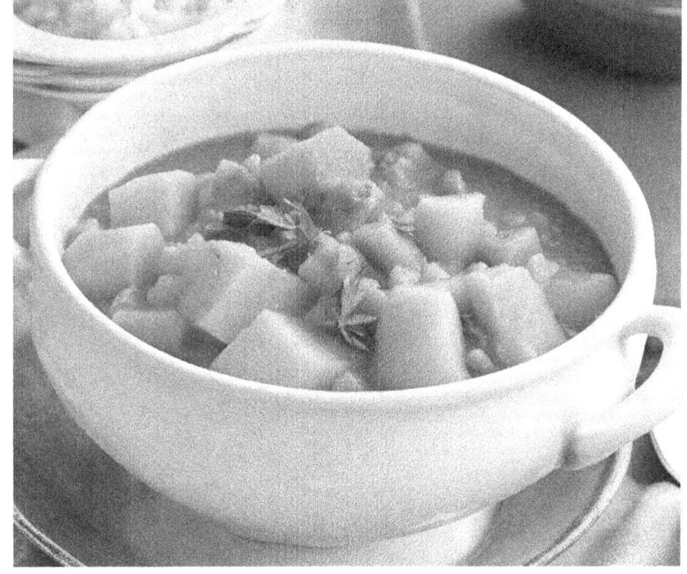

4. Roasted Root Vegetables

Ingredients:

- 2 medium sweet potatoes, peeled and cubed
- 2 medium parsnips, peeled and cubed
- 2 medium carrots, peeled and cubed
- 1 tablespoon olive oil
- 1 teaspoon dried rosemary
- 1 teaspoon dried thyme
- Fresh parsley for garnish

Instructions:

1. Preheat the oven to 400°F (200°C).
2. In a large bowl, toss the sweet potatoes, parsnips, and carrots with olive oil, dried rosemary, and thyme.
3. Spread the vegetables in a single layer on a baking sheet.
4. Roast for 25-30 minutes, or until the vegetables are tender and lightly browned, stirring halfway through.
5. Serve hot, garnished with fresh parsley.

Nutrition Info (Per Serving):

- Calories: 180
- Protein: 2g
- Carbohydrates: 35g
- Dietary Fiber: 7g
- Sugars: 12g
- Total Fat: 5g
- Saturated Fat: 0.5g
- Sodium: 60mg

Serves:

- **4 servings**

Cooking Time:

- **Total: 35 minutes**

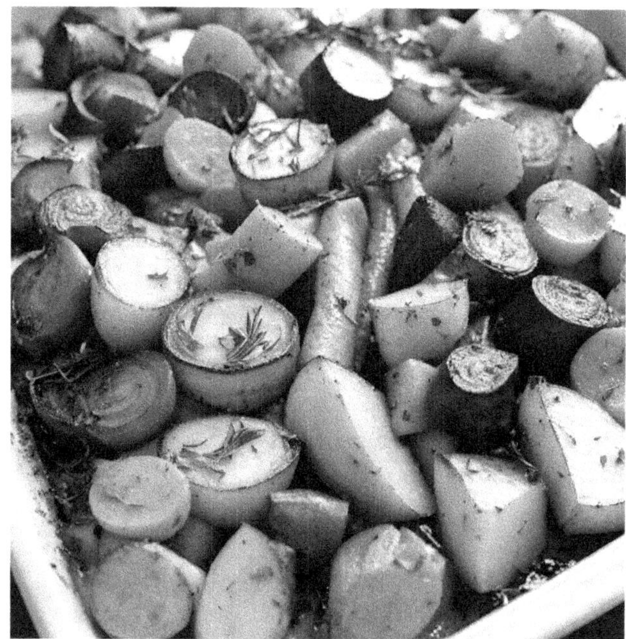

5. Parsleyed Corn

Ingredients:

- 4 ears of corn, husked
- 2 tablespoons olive oil
- 1/4 cup fresh parsley, chopped
- Fresh lemon wedges (if tolerated) for serving

Instructions:

1. Bring a large pot of water to a boil.
2. Add the corn and cook for 5-7 minutes until tender.
3. Remove the corn from the water and let cool slightly.
4. Brush the corn with olive oil and sprinkle with fresh parsley.
5. Serve with fresh lemon wedges (if tolerated).

Nutrition Info (Per Serving):

- Calories: 140
- Protein: 3g
- Carbohydrates: 21g
- Dietary Fiber: 3g
- Sugars: 6g
- Total Fat: 7g
- Saturated Fat: 1g
- Sodium: 20mg

Serves:

- 4 servings

Cooking Time:

- **Total: 10 minutes**

6. Kale and Potato Gratin

Ingredients:

- 4 medium potatoes, thinly sliced
- 2 cups fresh kale, chopped
- 1 cup unsweetened almond milk
- 1/2 cup low-fat shredded cheese (optional)
- 2 tablespoons olive oil
- 1 teaspoon dried thyme
- 1 teaspoon dried rosemary

Instructions:

1. Preheat the oven to 375°F (190°C).
2. Grease a baking dish with olive oil.
3. Layer half of the sliced potatoes in the bottom of the dish.
4. Spread the chopped kale evenly over the potatoes.
5. Layer the remaining sliced potatoes on top of the kale.
6. In a small bowl, mix the almond milk, dried thyme, and dried rosemary.
7. Pour the almond milk mixture over the layered potatoes and kale.
8. Sprinkle the shredded cheese on top (if using).
9. Cover with aluminum foil and bake for 40 minutes.
10. Remove the foil and bake for an additional 10-15 minutes, or until the top is golden and the potatoes are tender.
11. Serve hot.

Nutrition Info (Per Serving):

- Calories: 180
- Protein: 5g
- Carbohydrates: 28g
- Dietary Fiber: 4g
- Sugars: 3g
- Total Fat: 6g
- Saturated Fat: 1g
- Sodium: 150mg

Serves:

- 4 servings

Cooking Time:

- **Total: 55 minutes**

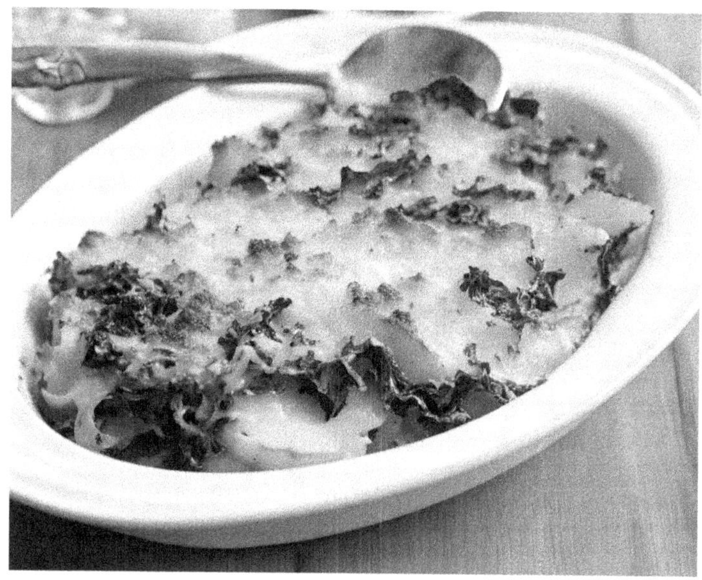

7. Baked Sweet Potato Fries

Ingredients:

- 2 large sweet potatoes, cut into thin fries
- 2 tablespoons olive oil
- 1 teaspoon dried thyme
- 1 teaspoon dried rosemary

Instructions:

1. Preheat the oven to 425°F (220°C).
2. In a large bowl, toss the sweet potato fries with olive oil, dried thyme, and dried rosemary.
3. Spread the fries in a single layer on a baking sheet lined with parchment paper.
4. Bake for 20-25 minutes, turning halfway through, until crispy and golden brown.
5. Serve hot.

Nutrition Info (Per Serving):

- Calories: 150
- Protein: 2g
- Carbohydrates: 28g
- Dietary Fiber: 4g
- Sugars: 7g
- Total Fat: 5g
- Saturated Fat: 1g
- Sodium: 20mg

Serves:

- **4 servings**

Cooking Time:

- **Total: 30 minutes**

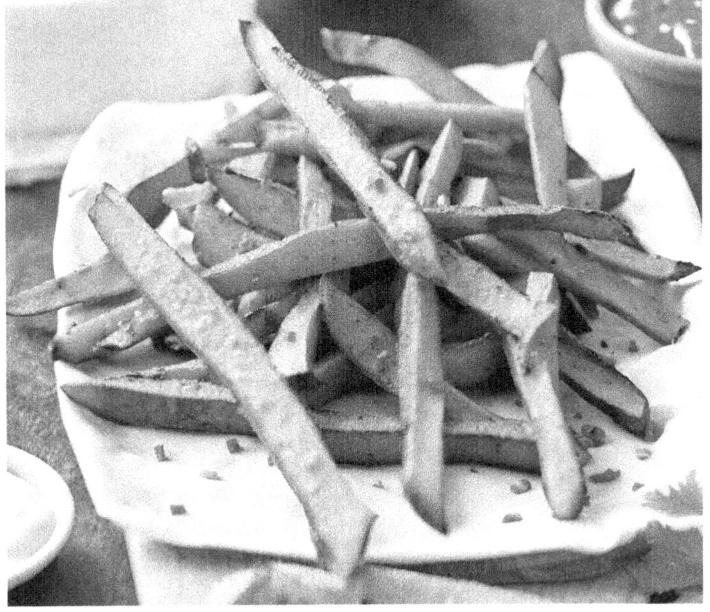

8. Steamed Beet Greens
Ingredients:

- 1 bunch beet greens, washed and chopped
- 1 tablespoon olive oil
- 1 teaspoon dried thyme
- Fresh lemon wedges (if tolerated) for serving

Instructions:

1. Bring a pot of water to a boil and place a steamer basket over it.
2. Add the chopped beet greens to the steamer basket and cover.
3. Steam for 3-5 minutes, or until the greens are tender.
4. Transfer the beet greens to a bowl and drizzle with olive oil.
5. Sprinkle with dried thyme and toss to coat.
6. Serve with fresh lemon wedges (if tolerated).

Nutrition Info (Per Serving):

- Calories: 60
- Protein: 2g
- Carbohydrates: 7g
- Dietary Fiber: 3g
- Sugars: 0g
- Total Fat: 3g
- Saturated Fat: 0.5g
- Sodium: 20mg

Serves:

- **4 servings**

Cooking Time:

- **Total: 10 minutes**

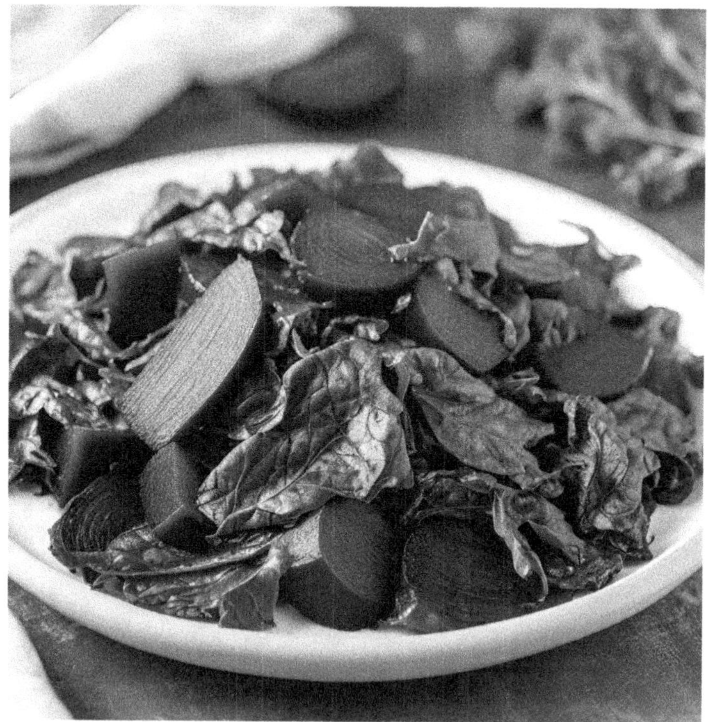

9. Eggplant Bake

Ingredients:

- 2 medium eggplants, sliced into rounds
- 2 cups unsweetened almond milk
- 1 cup low-fat shredded cheese (optional)
- 2 tablespoons olive oil
- 1 teaspoon dried oregano
- 1 teaspoon dried basil

Instructions:

1. Preheat the oven to 375°F (190°C).
2. Grease a baking dish with olive oil.
3. Layer the eggplant slices in the baking dish.
4. In a small bowl, mix the almond milk, dried oregano, and dried basil.
5. Pour the almond milk mixture over the eggplant slices.
6. Sprinkle the shredded cheese on top (if using).
7. Cover with aluminum foil and bake for 30 minutes.
8. Remove the foil and bake for an additional 10-15 minutes, or until the top is golden and the eggplant is tender.
9. Serve hot.

Nutrition Info (Per Serving):

- Calories: 160
- Protein: 4g
- Carbohydrates: 12g
- Dietary Fiber: 5g
- Sugars: 2g
- Total Fat: 10g
- Saturated Fat: 2g
- Sodium: 150mg

Serves:

- **4 servings**

Cooking Time:

- **Total: 45 minutes**

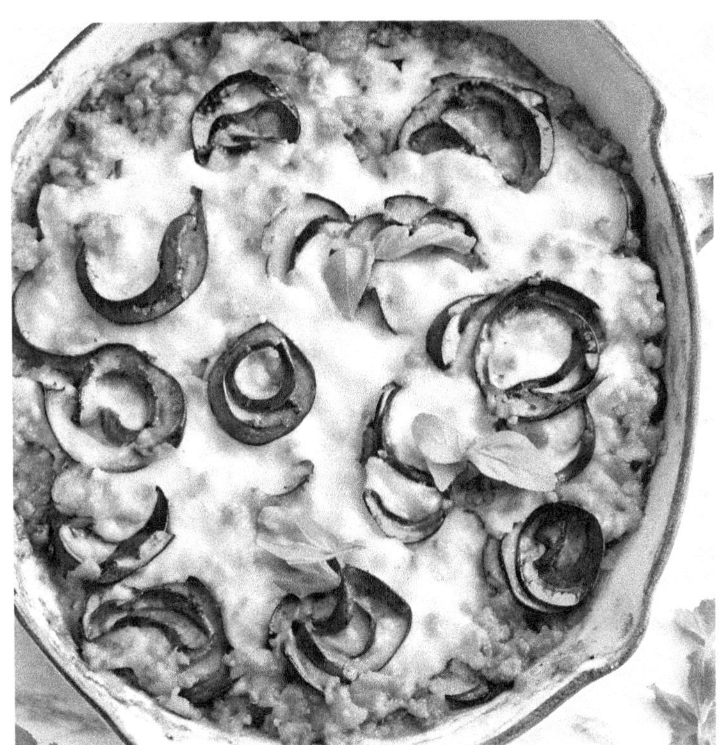

10. Celery Root Slaw

Ingredients:

- 1 medium celery root, peeled and shredded
- 2 medium carrots, shredded
- 1/4 cup plain yogurt (dairy or soy)
- 1 tablespoon olive oil
- 1 tablespoon honey
- 1 teaspoon dried dill

Instructions:

1. In a large bowl, combine the shredded celery root and shredded carrots.
2. In a small bowl, mix the yogurt, olive oil, honey, and dried dill.
3. Pour the dressing over the shredded vegetables and toss to coat.
4. Chill in the refrigerator for at least 30 minutes before serving.

Nutrition Info (Per Serving):

- Calories: 90
- Protein: 2g
- Carbohydrates: 14g
- Dietary Fiber: 4g
- Sugars: 8g
- Total Fat: 4g
- Saturated Fat: 0.5g
- Sodium: 60mg

Serves:

- **4 servings**

Cooking Time:

- **Total: 10 minutes (plus chilling time)**

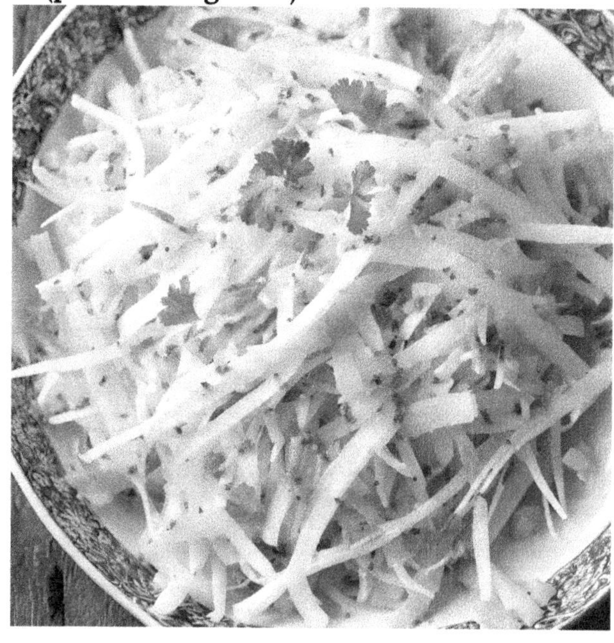

11. Stuffed Zucchini

Ingredients:

- 4 medium zucchinis
- 1 cup cooked quinoa
- 1/2 cup grated carrots
- 1/2 cup chopped spinach
- 1/4 cup grated low-fat cheese (optional)
- 1 tablespoon olive oil
- 1 teaspoon dried oregano

Instructions:

1. Preheat the oven to 375°F (190°C).
2. Cut the zucchinis in half lengthwise and scoop out the centers to create boats.
3. In a large bowl, mix the cooked quinoa, grated carrots, chopped spinach, olive oil, and dried oregano.
4. Stuff the zucchini boats with the quinoa mixture.
5. Place the stuffed zucchinis on a baking sheet and sprinkle with grated cheese (if using).
6. Bake for 25-30 minutes, or until the zucchinis are tender and the tops are golden.
7. Serve hot.

Nutrition Info (Per Serving):

- Calories: 150
- Protein: 5g
- Carbohydrates: 20g
- Dietary Fiber: 4g
- Sugars: 4g
- Total Fat: 6g
- Saturated Fat: 1g
- Sodium: 50mg

Serves:

- **4 servings**

Cooking Time:

- **Total: 35 minutes**

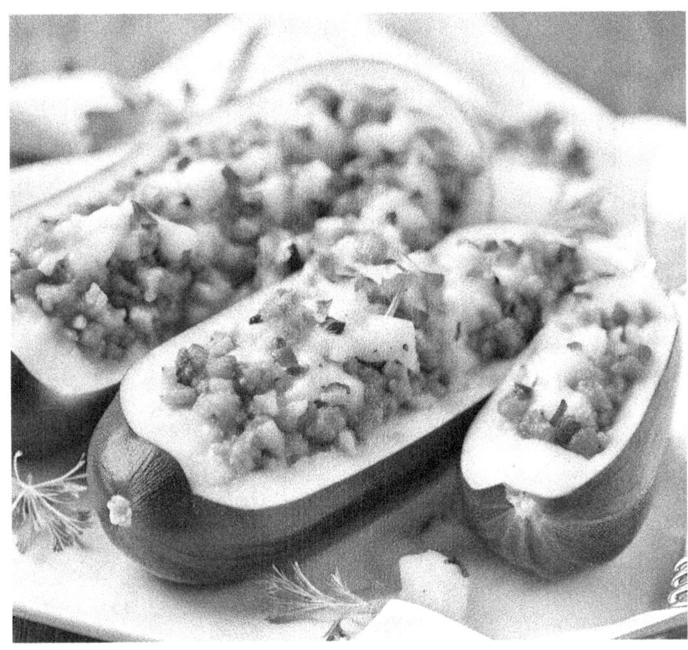

12. Braised Leeks

Ingredients:

- 4 large leeks, trimmed and cleaned
- 2 cups low-sodium vegetable broth
- 1 tablespoon olive oil
- 1 teaspoon dried thyme
- Fresh parsley for garnish

Instructions:

1. Preheat the oven to 350°F (175°C).
2. Cut the leeks in half lengthwise.
3. In a large oven-safe skillet, heat the olive oil over medium heat.
4. Add the leeks, cut side down, and cook for 3-4 minutes until lightly browned.
5. Pour in the vegetable broth and sprinkle with dried thyme.
6. Cover the skillet and transfer to the oven. Braise for 25-30 minutes, or until the leeks are tender.
7. Serve hot, garnished with fresh parsley.

Nutrition Info (Per Serving):

- Calories: 90
- Protein: 2g
- Carbohydrates: 14g
- Dietary Fiber: 3g
- Sugars: 4g
- Total Fat: 4g
- Saturated Fat: 0.5g
- Sodium: 150mg

Serves:

- **4 servings**

Cooking Time:

- **Total: 35 minutes**

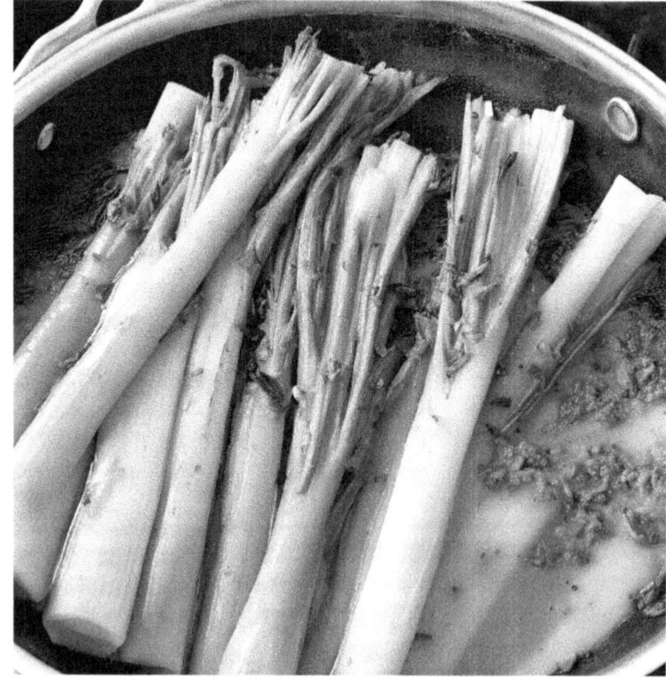

13. Fennel and Apple Salad

Ingredients:

- 1 large fennel bulb, thinly sliced
- 2 medium apples, thinly sliced
- 1/4 cup walnuts, chopped
- 1/4 cup plain yogurt (dairy or soy)
- 1 tablespoon olive oil
- 1 tablespoon honey
- 1 teaspoon dried dill

Instructions:

1. In a large bowl, combine the sliced fennel, sliced apples, and chopped walnuts.
2. In a small bowl, mix the yogurt, olive oil, honey, and dried dill.
3. Pour the dressing over the salad and toss to coat.
4. Chill in the refrigerator for at least 15 minutes before serving.

Nutrition Info (Per Serving):

- Calories: 120
- Protein: 2g
- Carbohydrates: 18g
- Dietary Fiber: 4g
- Sugars: 10g
- Total Fat: 6g
- Saturated Fat: 0.5g
- Sodium: 40mg

Serves:

- **4 servings**

Cooking Time:

- **Total: 20 minutes (plus chilling time)**

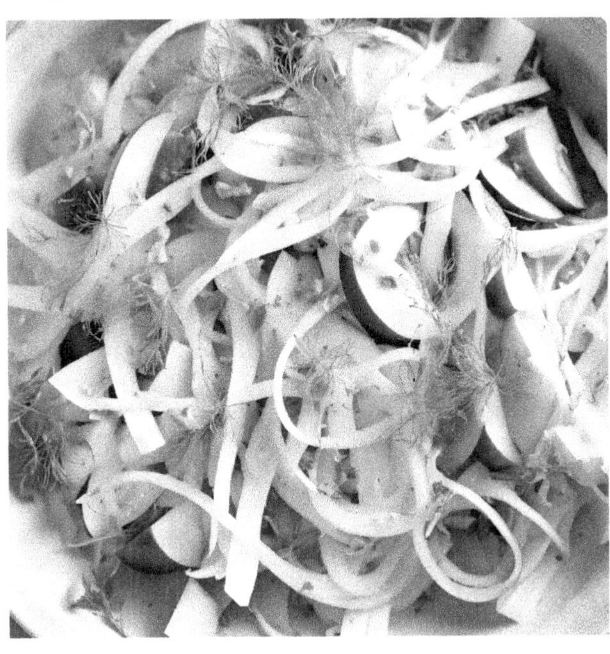

14. Creamy Potato Soup

Ingredients:

- 4 medium potatoes, peeled and diced
- 4 cups low-sodium vegetable broth
- 1 cup unsweetened almond milk
- 2 medium carrots, diced
- 2 celery stalks, diced
- 1 tablespoon olive oil
- 1 teaspoon dried thyme
- Fresh parsley for garnish

Instructions:

1. In a large pot, heat the olive oil over medium heat.
2. Add the diced potatoes, carrots, and celery, and cook for 5 minutes until slightly softened.
3. Add the vegetable broth and dried thyme, and bring to a boil.
4. Reduce heat to low and simmer for 15-20 minutes, or until the vegetables are tender.
5. Using an immersion blender, blend the soup until smooth.
6. Stir in the almond milk and cook for an additional 5 minutes.
7. Serve hot, garnished with fresh parsley.

Nutrition Info (Per Serving):

- Calories: 150
- Protein: 3g
- Carbohydrates: 28g
- Dietary Fiber: 4g
- Sugars: 4g
- Total Fat: 4g
- Saturated Fat: 0.5g
- Sodium: 120mg

Serves:

- **4 servings**

Cooking Time:

- **Total: 30 minutes**

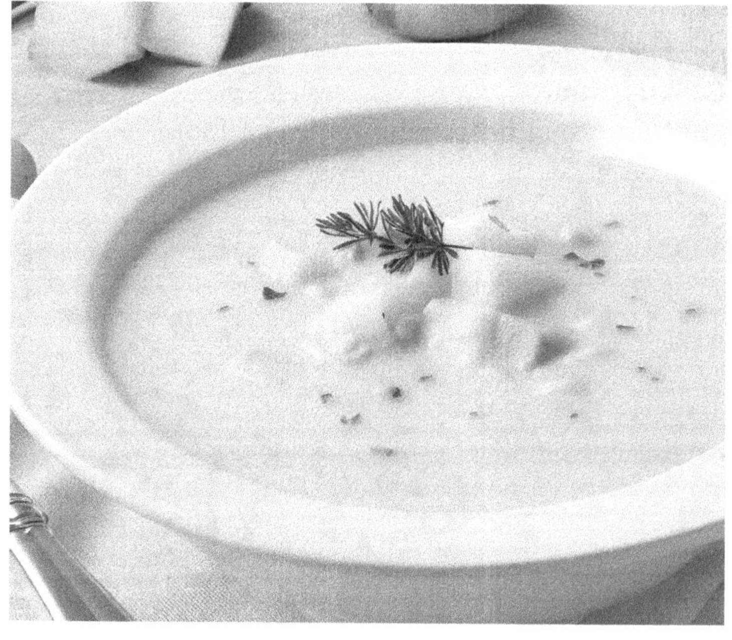

15. Roasted Brussels Sprouts

Ingredients:

- 1 pound Brussels sprouts, trimmed and halved
- 2 tablespoons olive oil
- 1 teaspoon dried rosemary
- 1 teaspoon dried thyme
- Fresh lemon wedges (if tolerated) for serving

Instructions:

1. Preheat the oven to 400°F (200°C).
2. In a large bowl, toss the Brussels sprouts with olive oil, dried rosemary, and thyme.
3. Spread the Brussels sprouts in a single layer on a baking sheet lined with parchment paper.
4. Roast for 20-25 minutes, or until tender and lightly browned, stirring halfway through.
5. Serve hot with fresh lemon wedges (if tolerated).

Nutrition Info (Per Serving):

- Calories: 120
- Protein: 4g
- Carbohydrates: 12g
- Dietary Fiber: 5g
- Sugars: 3g
- Total Fat: 7g
- Saturated Fat: 1g
- Sodium: 40mg

Serves:

- **4 servings**

Cooking Time:

- **Total: 30 minutes**

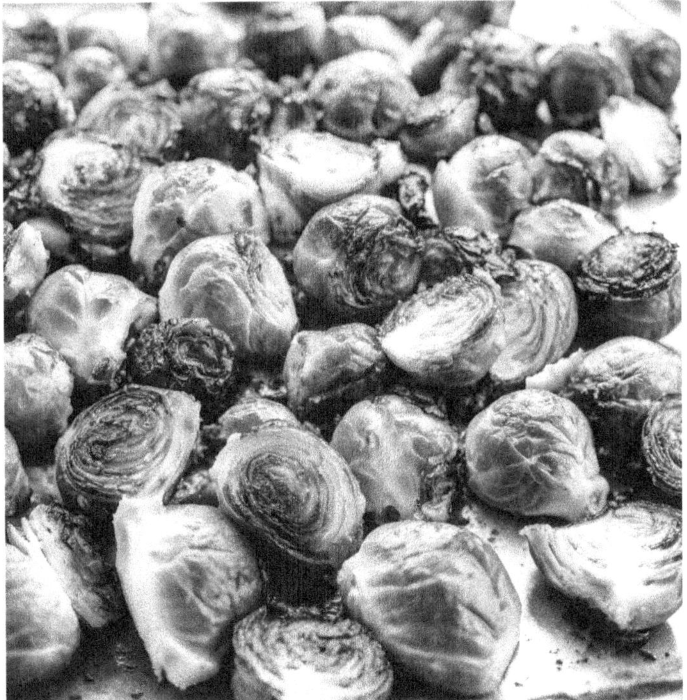

16. Baked Parsnips

Ingredients:

- 4 large parsnips, peeled and cut into sticks
- 2 tablespoons olive oil
- 1 teaspoon dried thyme
- 1 teaspoon dried rosemary

Instructions:

1. Preheat the oven to 400°F (200°C).
2. In a large bowl, toss the parsnip sticks with olive oil, dried thyme, and rosemary.
3. Spread the parsnips in a single layer on a baking sheet lined with parchment paper.
4. Bake for 25-30 minutes, or until tender and golden brown, stirring halfway through.
5. Serve hot.

Nutrition Info (Per Serving):

- Calories: 120
- Protein: 2g
- Carbohydrates: 22g
- Dietary Fiber: 6g
- Sugars: 6g
- Total Fat: 5g
- Saturated Fat: 0.5g
- Sodium: 20mg

Serves:

- **4 servings**

Cooking Time:

- **Total: 35 minutes**

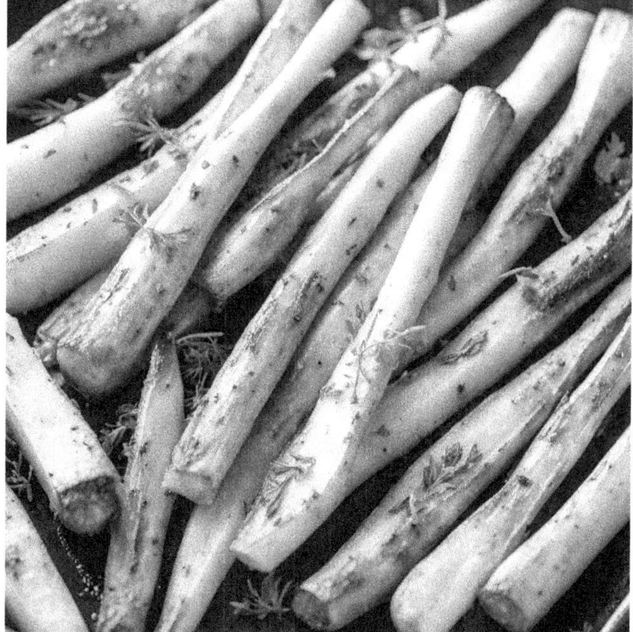

17. Turnip and Leek Soup

Ingredients:

- 4 large turnips, peeled and diced
- 2 large leeks, trimmed and sliced
- 4 cups low-sodium vegetable broth
- 1 cup unsweetened almond milk
- 1 tablespoon olive oil
- 1 teaspoon dried thyme
- Fresh parsley for garnish

Instructions:

1. In a large pot, heat the olive oil over medium heat.
2. Add the sliced leeks and cook for 3-4 minutes until softened.
3. Add the diced turnips, vegetable broth, and dried thyme, and bring to a boil.
4. Reduce heat to low and simmer for 15-20 minutes, or until the turnips are tender.
5. Using an immersion blender, blend the soup until smooth.
6. Stir in the almond milk and cook for an additional 5 minutes.
7. Serve hot, garnished with fresh parsley.

Nutrition Info (Per Serving):

- Calories: 110
- Protein: 2g
- Carbohydrates: 20g
- Dietary Fiber: 4g
- Sugars: 6g
- Total Fat: 4g
- Saturated Fat: 0.5g
- Sodium: 120mg

Serves:

- **4 servings**

Cooking Time:

- **Total: 30 minutes**

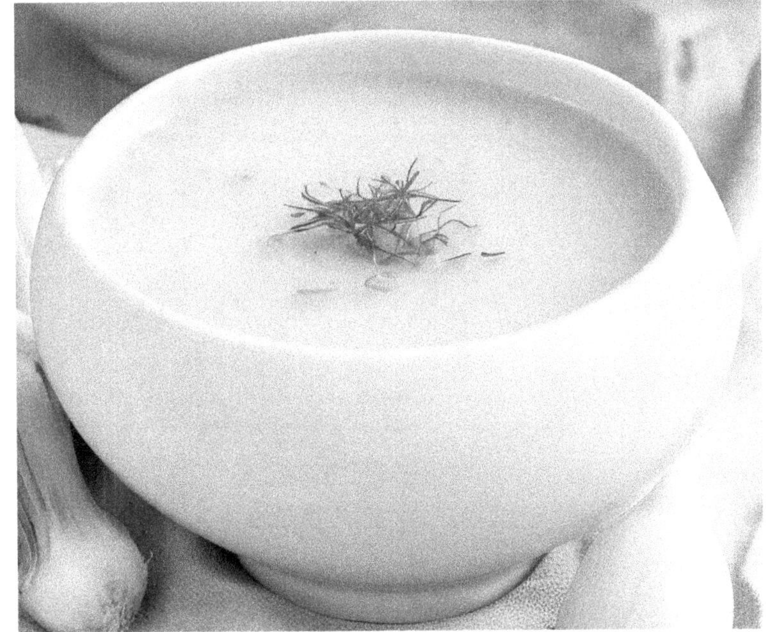

18. Rutabaga Mash

Ingredients:

- 4 large rutabagas, peeled and cubed
- 1/2 cup unsweetened almond milk
- 2 tablespoons unsalted butter
- 1 teaspoon dried thyme

Instructions:

1. In a large pot, bring water to a boil.
2. Add the cubed rutabagas and cook for 20-25 minutes, or until tender.
3. Drain the rutabagas and return them to the pot.
4. Add the almond milk, butter, and dried thyme.
5. Mash until smooth and creamy.
6. Serve hot.

Nutrition Info (Per Serving):

- Calories: 140
- Protein: 2g
- Carbohydrates: 21g
- Dietary Fiber: 5g
- Sugars: 8g
- Total Fat: 6g
- Saturated Fat: 2g
- Sodium: 40mg

Serves:

- **4 servings**

Cooking Time:

- **Total: 30 minutes**

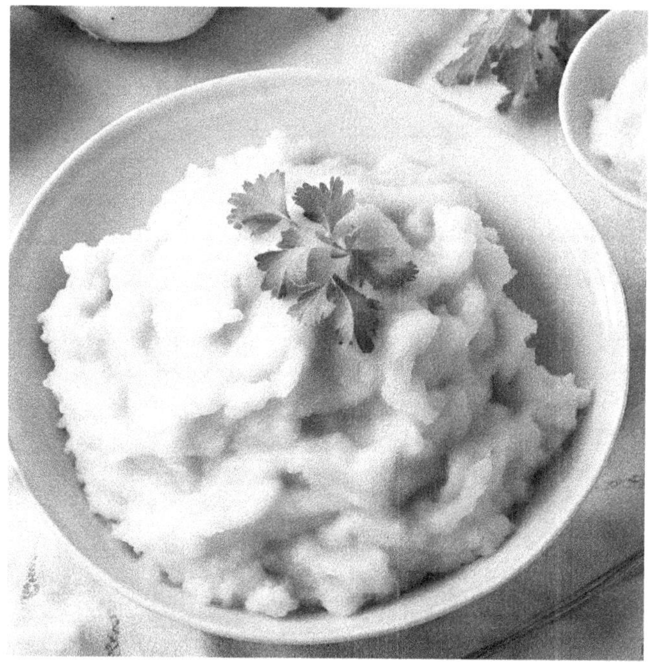

19. Squash and Apple Soup

Ingredients:

- 2 medium butternut squash, peeled, seeded, and cubed
- 2 large apples, peeled and diced
- 4 cups low-sodium vegetable broth
- 1 cup unsweetened almond milk
- 1 tablespoon olive oil
- 1 teaspoon dried sage
- Fresh parsley for garnish

Instructions:

1. In a large pot, heat the olive oil over medium heat.
2. Add the cubed squash and diced apples, and cook for 5 minutes until slightly softened.
3. Add the vegetable broth and dried sage, and bring to a boil.
4. Reduce heat to low and simmer for 20-25 minutes, or until the squash is tender.
5. Using an immersion blender, blend the soup until smooth.
6. Stir in the almond milk and cook for an additional 5 minutes.
7. Serve hot, garnished with fresh parsley.

Nutrition Info (Per Serving):

- Calories: 160
- Protein: 2g
- Carbohydrates: 35g
- Dietary Fiber: 7g
- Sugars: 15g
- Total Fat: 4g
- Saturated Fat: 0.5g
- Sodium: 120mg

Serves:

- **4 servings**

Cooking Time:

- **Total: 35 minutes**

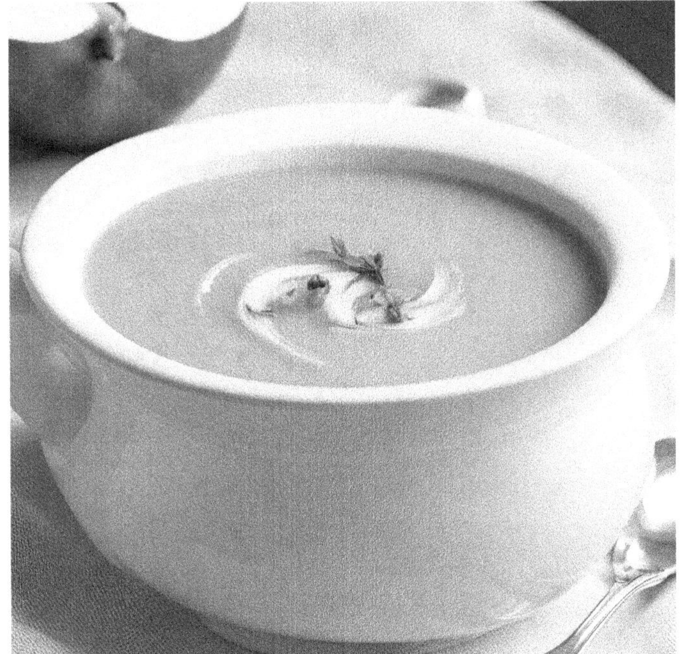

20. Herbed New Potatoes

Ingredients:

- 1 pound new potatoes, halved
- 2 tablespoons olive oil
- 1 teaspoon dried rosemary
- 1 teaspoon dried thyme
- Fresh parsley for garnish

Instructions:

1. Preheat the oven to 400°F (200°C).
2. In a large bowl, toss the halved new potatoes with olive oil, dried rosemary, and thyme.
3. Spread the potatoes in a single layer on a baking sheet lined with parchment paper.
4. Roast for 25-30 minutes, or until tender and golden brown, stirring halfway through.
5. Serve hot, garnished with fresh parsley.

Nutrition Info (Per Serving):

- Calories: 160
- Protein: 2g
- Carbohydrates: 28g
- Dietary Fiber: 4g
- Sugars: 2g
- Total Fat: 5g
- Saturated Fat: 0.5g
- Sodium: 20mg

Serves:

- **4 servings**

Cooking Time:

- **Total: 35 minutes**

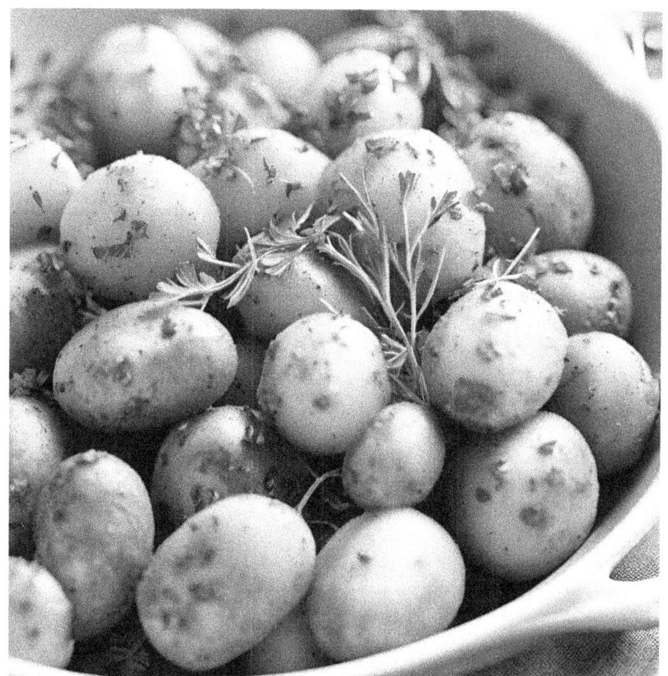

21. Steamed Artichokes

Ingredients:

- 4 large artichokes
- 1 lemon, cut into wedges (if tolerated)
- 2 tablespoons olive oil
- 1 teaspoon dried thyme

Instructions:

1. Trim the stems of the artichokes and remove the tough outer leaves.
2. Cut off the top quarter of each artichoke.
3. Fill a large pot with about 2 inches of water and bring to a boil.
4. Place a steamer basket in the pot and add the artichokes, cut side up.
5. Drizzle the artichokes with olive oil and sprinkle with dried thyme.
6. Cover and steam for 25-30 minutes, or until the leaves are tender and easily pull away.
7. Serve hot with lemon wedges (if tolerated).

Nutrition Info (Per Serving):

- Calories: 110
- Protein: 3g
- Carbohydrates: 14g
- Dietary Fiber: 7g
- Sugars: 1g
- Total Fat: 6g
- Saturated Fat: 1g
- Sodium: 75mg

Serves:

- 4 servings

Cooking Time:

- Total: 35 minutes

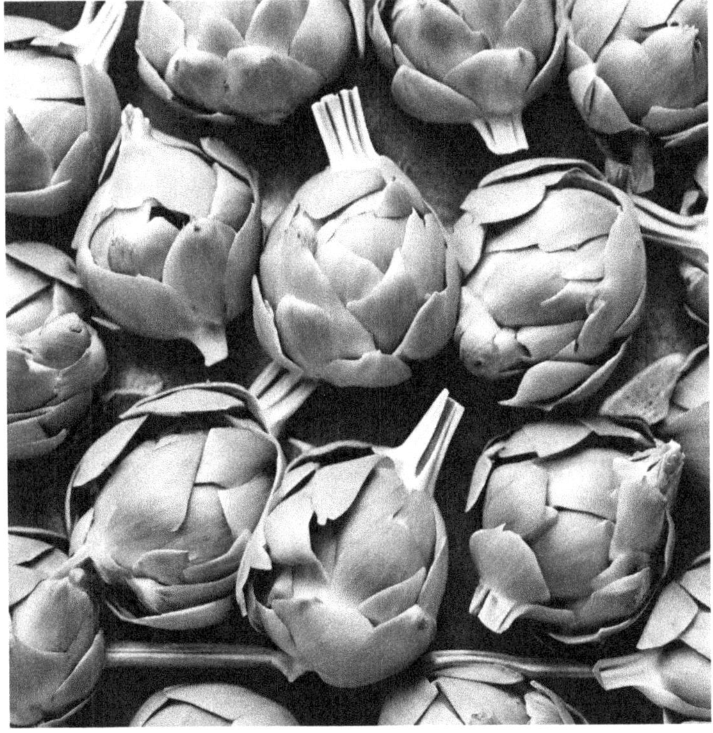

22. Beetroot and Carrot Salad

Ingredients:

- 2 large beetroots, peeled and grated
- 2 large carrots, peeled and grated
- 1/4 cup chopped fresh parsley
- 2 tablespoons olive oil
- 1 tablespoon lemon juice (if tolerated)
- 1 teaspoon dried dill

Instructions:

1. In a large bowl, combine the grated beetroots, grated carrots, and chopped parsley.
2. In a small bowl, whisk together the olive oil, lemon juice (if tolerated), and dried dill.
3. Pour the dressing over the salad and toss to coat.
4. Chill in the refrigerator for at least 15 minutes before serving.

Nutrition Info (Per Serving):

- Calories: 120
- Protein: 2g
- Carbohydrates: 15g
- Dietary Fiber: 4g
- Sugars: 9g
- Total Fat: 7g
- Saturated Fat: 1g
- Sodium: 50mg

Serves:

- **4 servings**

Cooking Time:

- **Total: 20 minutes (plus chilling time)**

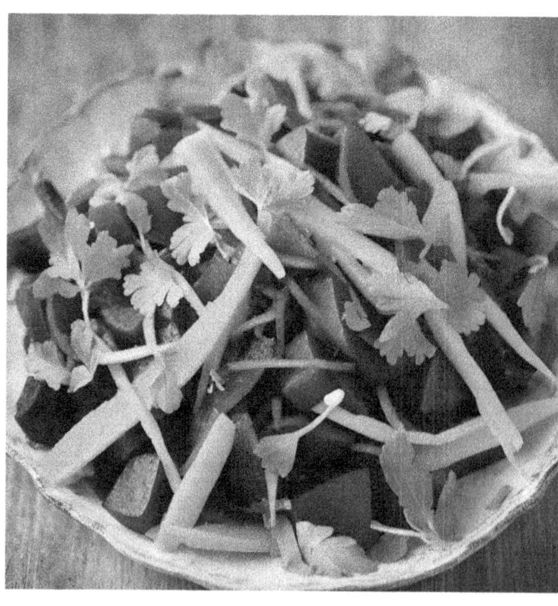

23. Green Beans Almondine

Ingredients:

- 1 pound fresh green beans, trimmed
- 1/4 cup sliced almonds
- 2 tablespoons olive oil
- 1 teaspoon dried thyme
- Fresh lemon wedges (if tolerated) for serving

Instructions:

1. Bring a large pot of water to a boil.
2. Add the green beans and cook for 3-4 minutes until tender-crisp.
3. Drain the green beans and set aside.
4. In a large skillet, heat the olive oil over medium heat.
5. Add the sliced almonds and cook for 2-3 minutes until golden brown.
6. Add the green beans to the skillet and toss to coat with the almonds and olive oil.
7. Sprinkle with dried thyme.
8. Serve hot with fresh lemon wedges (if tolerated).

Nutrition Info (Per Serving):

- Calories: 120
- Protein: 3g
- Carbohydrates: 10g
- Dietary Fiber: 4g
- Sugars: 4g
- Total Fat: 9g
- Saturated Fat: 1g
- Sodium: 15mg

Serves:

- **4 servings**

Cooking Time:

- **Total: 15 minutes**

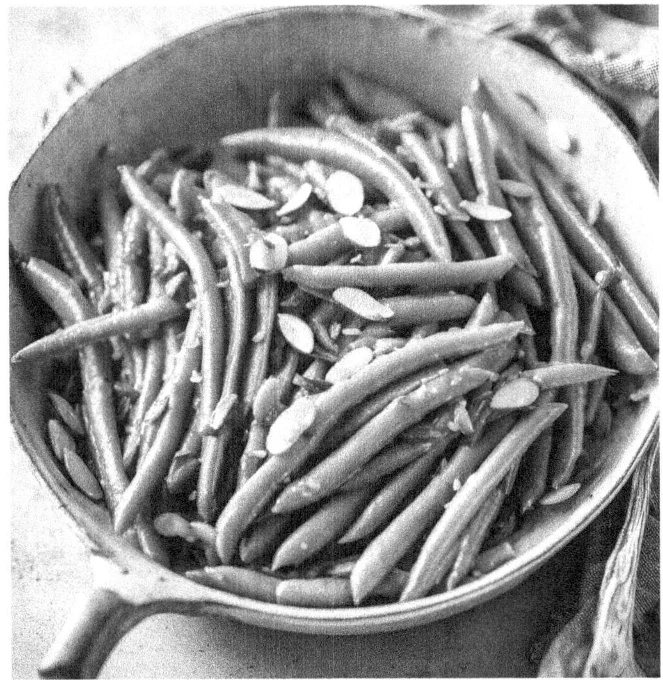

24. Pumpkin Porridge

Ingredients:

- 2 cups pureed pumpkin (canned or fresh)
- 1 cup rolled oats
- 3 cups unsweetened almond milk
- 1 tablespoon honey
- 1 teaspoon ground cinnamon
- 1/2 teaspoon ground nutmeg

Instructions:

1. In a large pot, combine the pureed pumpkin, rolled oats, and almond milk.
2. Bring to a boil over medium heat, then reduce heat to low and simmer for 10-15 minutes, stirring occasionally, until the oats are tender.
3. Stir in the honey, ground cinnamon, and ground nutmeg.
4. Serve hot.

Nutrition Info (Per Serving):

- Calories: 180
- Protein: 4g
- Carbohydrates: 36g
- Dietary Fiber: 6g
- Sugars: 8g
- Total Fat: 3g
- Saturated Fat: 0.5g
- Sodium: 60mg

Serves:

- **4 servings**

Cooking Time:

- **Total: 20 minutes**

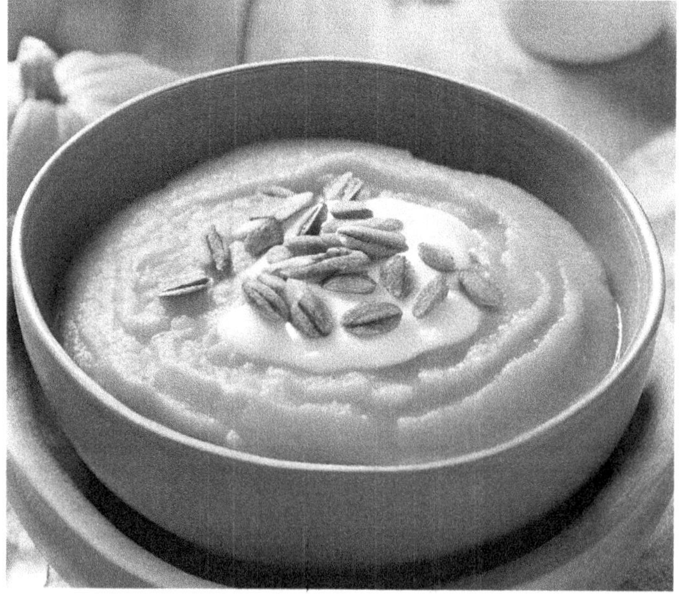

Desserts

1. Apple Ginger Tea
Ingredients:
- 2 large apples, sliced
- 1-inch piece fresh ginger, peeled and sliced
- 4 cups water
- 1 tablespoon honey (optional)
- 1 cinnamon stick

Instructions:
1. In a large pot, combine the sliced apples, ginger, water, and cinnamon stick.
2. Bring to a boil over medium heat, then reduce heat to low and simmer for 20 minutes.
3. Strain the tea into cups.
4. Stir in honey (if using) before serving.

Nutrition Info (Per Serving):
- Calories: 40
- Protein: 0g
- Carbohydrates: 10g
- Dietary Fiber: 1g
- Sugars: 8g
- Total Fat: 0g
- Saturated Fat: 0g
- Sodium: 0mg

Serves:
- **4 servings**

Cooking Time:
- **Total: 25 minutes**

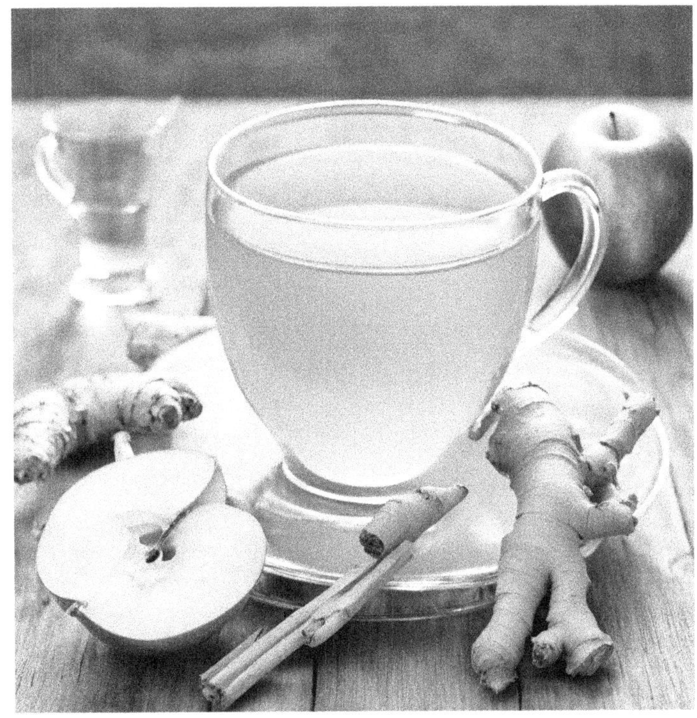

2. Watermelon Juice

Ingredients:

- 4 cups watermelon, cubed and seeds removed
- 1 tablespoon fresh mint leaves
- 1 tablespoon lemon juice (if tolerated)
- 1 cup water

Instructions:

1. In a blender, combine the watermelon cubes, fresh mint leaves, lemon juice (if tolerated), and water.
2. Blend until smooth.
3. Strain the juice through a fine mesh sieve to remove any pulp.
4. Serve chilled.

Nutrition Info (Per Serving):

- Calories: 40
- Protein: 1g
- Carbohydrates: 10g
- Dietary Fiber: 0g
- Sugars: 8g
- Total Fat: 0g
- Saturated Fat: 0g
- Sodium: 0mg

Serves:

- **4 servings**

Cooking Time:

- **Total: 10 minutes**

3. Pear Nectar

Ingredients:

- 4 ripe pears, peeled, cored, and chopped
- 2 cups water
- 1 tablespoon honey (optional)

Instructions:

1. In a blender, combine the chopped pears and water.
2. Blend until smooth.
3. Strain the mixture through a fine mesh sieve to remove any pulp.
4. Stir in honey (if using) before serving.
5. Serve chilled.

Nutrition Info (Per Serving):

- Calories: 60
- Protein: 0g
- Carbohydrates: 16g
- Dietary Fiber: 3g
- Sugars: 12g
- Total Fat: 0g
- Saturated Fat: 0g
- Sodium: 0mg

Serves:

- **4 servings**

Cooking Time:

- **Total: 10 minutes**

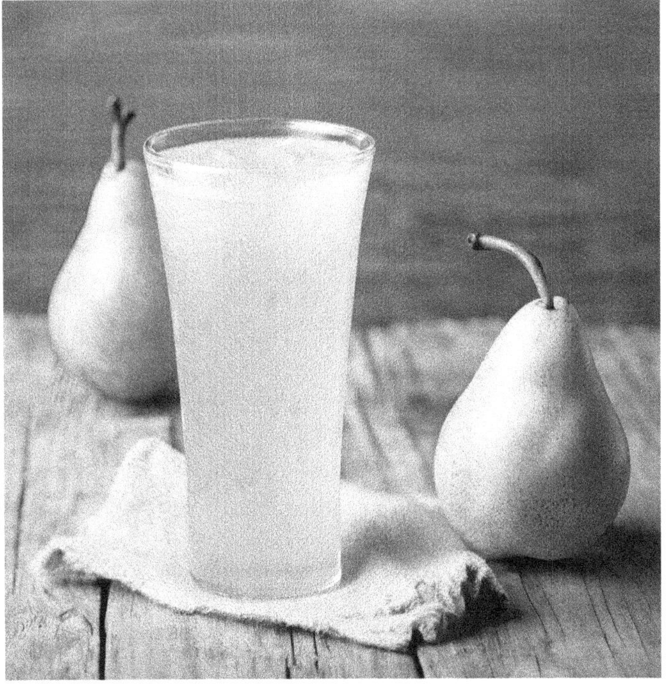

4. Oat Milk Latte

Ingredients:

- 2 cups oat milk
- 1 cup brewed decaffeinated coffee
- 1 tablespoon honey (optional)
- 1/2 teaspoon ground cinnamon

Instructions:

1. In a small saucepan, heat the oat milk over medium heat until hot but not boiling.
2. Brew a cup of decaffeinated coffee.
3. Pour the hot oat milk and decaffeinated coffee into a blender.
4. Add honey (if using) and ground cinnamon.
5. Blend until frothy.
6. Pour into mugs and serve hot.

Nutrition Info (Per Serving):

- Calories: 70
- Protein: 1g
- Carbohydrates: 15g
- Dietary Fiber: 1g
- Sugars: 8g
- Total Fat: 2g
- Saturated Fat: 0g
- Sodium: 50mg

Serves:

- **2 servings**

Cooking Time:

- **Total: 10 minutes**

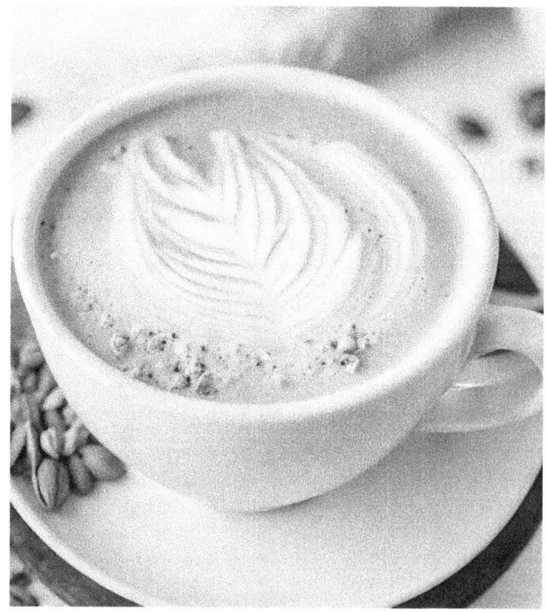

5. Coconut Rice Dessert

Ingredients:

- 1 cup jasmine rice
- 2 cups unsweetened coconut milk
- 1/4 cup honey
- 1 teaspoon vanilla extract
- 1/4 cup shredded coconut (optional)

Instructions:

1. In a medium saucepan, combine the jasmine rice and coconut milk.
2. Bring to a boil over medium heat, then reduce heat to low and simmer for 20 minutes, or until the rice is tender and the liquid is absorbed.
3. Stir in the honey and vanilla extract.
4. Serve warm, topped with shredded coconut (if using).

Nutrition Info (Per Serving):

- Calories: 180
- Protein: 3g
- Carbohydrates: 35g
- Dietary Fiber: 1g
- Sugars: 15g
- Total Fat: 3g
- Saturated Fat: 2g
- Sodium: 10mg

Serves:

- **4 servings**

Cooking Time:

- **Total: 25 minutes**

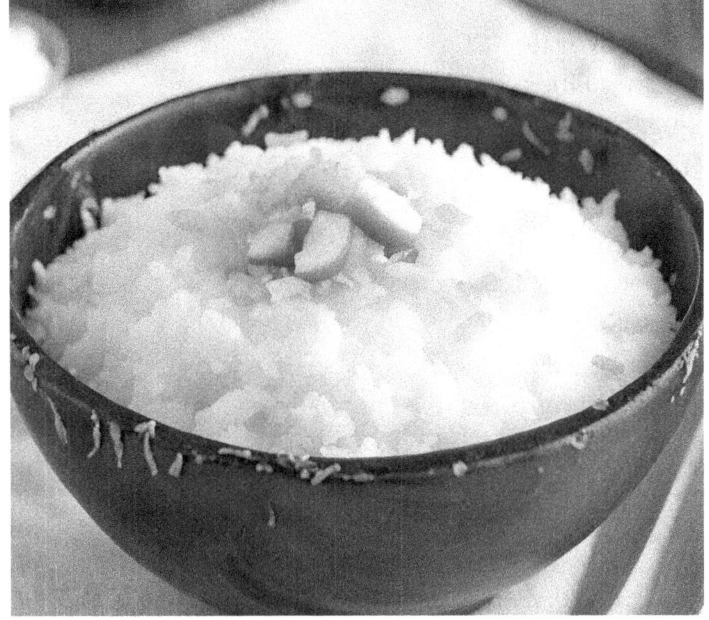

6. Pumpkin Custard

Ingredients:

- 1 cup pureed pumpkin (canned or fresh)
- 1 cup unsweetened almond milk
- 2 large eggs
- 1/4 cup honey
- 1 teaspoon ground cinnamon
- 1/2 teaspoon ground nutmeg

Instructions:

1. Preheat the oven to 350°F (175°C).
2. In a large bowl, whisk together the pureed pumpkin, almond milk, eggs, honey, ground cinnamon, and ground nutmeg until smooth.
3. Pour the mixture into ramekins.
4. Place the ramekins in a baking dish and add hot water to the dish to come halfway up the sides of the ramekins.
5. Bake for 30-35 minutes, or until the custards are set.
6. Serve chilled.

Nutrition Info (Per Serving):

- Calories: 120
- Protein: 4g
- Carbohydrates: 20g
- Dietary Fiber: 2g
- Sugars: 15g
- Total Fat: 3g
- Saturated Fat: 0.5g
- Sodium: 40mg

Serves:

- **4 servings**

Cooking Time:

- **Total: 40 minutes**

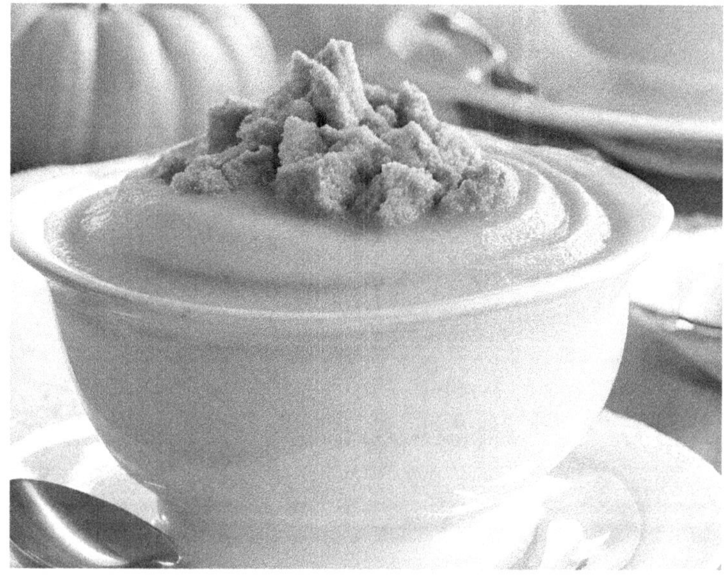

7. Banana Almond Smoothie

Ingredients:

- 2 ripe bananas
- 1 cup unsweetened almond milk
- 1/4 cup almond butter
- 1 tablespoon honey
- 1/2 teaspoon ground cinnamon

Instructions:

1. In a blender, combine the bananas, almond milk, almond butter, honey, and ground cinnamon.
2. Blend until smooth.
3. Serve chilled.

Nutrition Info (Per Serving):

- Calories: 150
- Protein: 3g
- Carbohydrates: 28g
- Dietary Fiber: 4g
- Sugars: 18g
- Total Fat: 5g
- Saturated Fat: 0.5g
- Sodium: 30mg

Serves:

- **2 servings**

Cooking Time:

- **Total: 5 minutes**

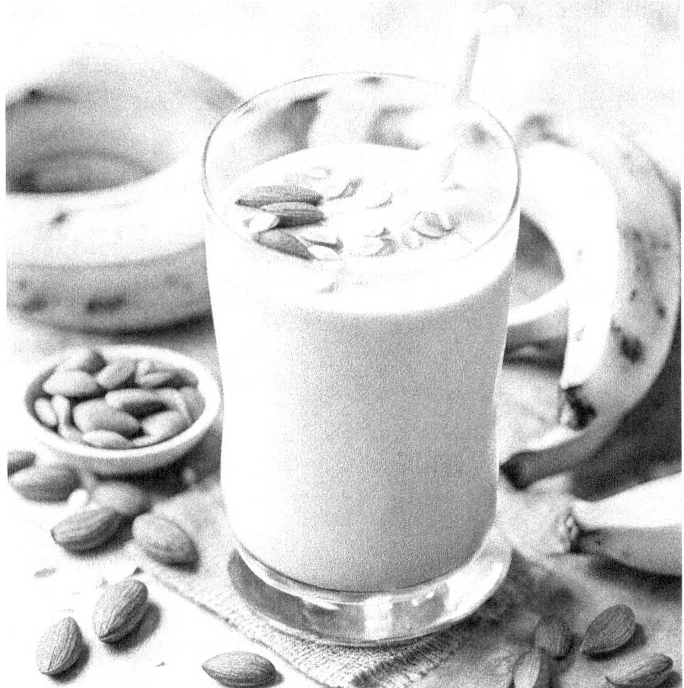

8. Blueberry Oat Smoothie

Ingredients:

- 1 cup fresh or frozen blueberries
- 1/2 cup rolled oats
- 1 cup unsweetened almond milk
- 1 tablespoon honey
- 1/2 teaspoon ground cinnamon
- 1/2 teaspoon vanilla extract

Instructions:

1. In a blender, combine the blueberries, rolled oats, almond milk, honey, ground cinnamon, and vanilla extract.
2. Blend until smooth.
3. Pour into glasses and serve chilled.

Nutrition Info (Per Serving):

- Calories: 180
- Protein: 4g
- Carbohydrates: 35g
- Dietary Fiber: 6g
- Sugars: 15g
- Total Fat: 3g
- Saturated Fat: 0g
- Sodium: 50mg

Serves:

- **2 servings**

Cooking Time:

- **Total: 5 minutes**

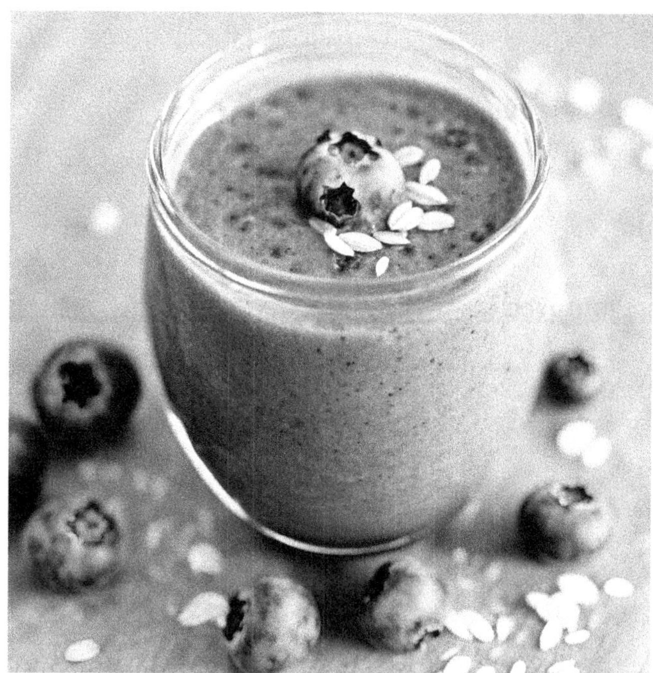

9. Peach Smoothie

Ingredients:

- 2 ripe peaches, peeled and sliced
- 1 cup unsweetened almond milk
- 1/2 cup plain yogurt (dairy or soy)
- 1 tablespoon honey
- 1/2 teaspoon ground cinnamon

Instructions:

1. In a blender, combine the sliced peaches, almond milk, yogurt, honey, and ground cinnamon.
2. Blend until smooth.
3. Pour into glasses and serve chilled.

Nutrition Info (Per Serving):

- Calories: 150
- Protein: 4g
- Carbohydrates: 28g
- Dietary Fiber: 3g
- Sugars: 20g
- Total Fat: 3g
- Saturated Fat: 0.5g
- Sodium: 60mg

Serves:

- **2 servings**

Cooking Time:

- **Total: 5 minutes**

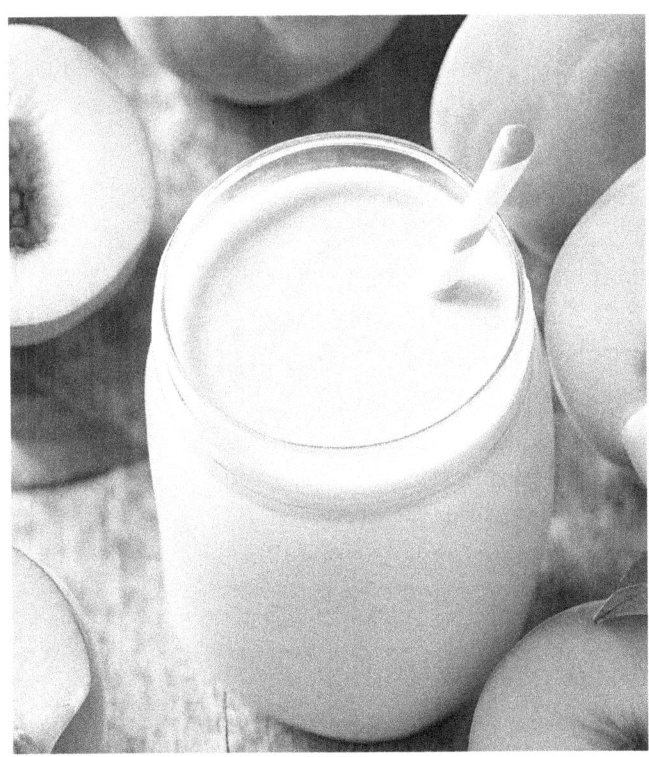

10-WEEK MEAL PLAN

Week 1

Monday
- Breakfast: Blueberry Oat Smoothie
- Lunch: Mushroom and Barley Soup
- Dinner: Baked Chicken with Barley
- Snack: Apple Ginger Tea

Tuesday
- Breakfast: Pear Nectar
- Lunch: Squash Stew
- Dinner: Turkey Quinoa Pilaf
- Snack: Watermelon Juice

Wednesday
- Breakfast: Banana Almond Smoothie
- Lunch: Steamed Beet Greens
- Dinner: Chicken with Mashed Potatoes
- Snack: Oat Milk Latte

Thursday
- Breakfast: Peach Smoothie
- Lunch: Stuffed Zucchini
- Dinner: Turkey and Sweet Potato Stew
- Snack: Pumpkin Custard

Friday
- Breakfast: Coconut Rice Dessert
- Lunch: Green Beans Almondine
- Dinner: Oven-Roasted Turkey Breast
- Snack: Apple Ginger Tea

Saturday
- Breakfast: Blueberry Oat Smoothie
- Lunch: Beetroot and Carrot Salad
- Dinner: Turkey Apple Burgers
- Snack: Pear Nectar

Sunday
- Breakfast: Pumpkin Porridge
- Lunch: Braised Leeks
- Dinner: Chicken Porridge
- Snack: Banana Almond Smoothie

Week 2

Monday
- Breakfast: Watermelon Juice
- Lunch: Roasted Root Vegetables
- Dinner: Grilled Turkey Breast
- Snack: Peach Smoothie

Tuesday
- Breakfast: Apple Ginger Tea
- Lunch: Steamed Artichokes
- Dinner: Turkey and Zucchini Patties
- Snack: Coconut Rice Dessert

Wednesday
- Breakfast: Pear Nectar
- Lunch: Celery Root Slaw
- Dinner: Chicken and Vegetable Skewers
- Snack: Oat Milk Latte

Thursday
- Breakfast: Blueberry Oat Smoothie
- Lunch: Squash and Apple Soup
- Dinner: Slow Cooker Chicken with Carrots
- Snack: Pumpkin Custard

Friday
- Breakfast: Banana Almond Smoothie
- Lunch: Stuffed Zucchini
- Dinner: Baked Turkey Meatloaf
- Snack: Watermelon Juice

Saturday
- Breakfast: Pumpkin Porridge
- Lunch: Fennel and Apple Salad
- Dinner: Chicken Rice Paper Rolls
- Snack: Apple Ginger Tea

Sunday
- Breakfast: Peach Smoothie
- Lunch: Herbed New Potatoes
- Dinner: Roast Turkey with Squash
- Snack: Pear Nectar

Week 3

Monday
- Breakfast: Coconut Rice Dessert
- Lunch: Green Beans Almondine
- Dinner: Chicken Pea Soup
- Snack: Blueberry Oat Smoothie

Tuesday

- Breakfast: Banana Almond Smoothie
- Lunch: Roasted Brussels Sprouts
- Dinner: Turkey Pilaf
- Snack: Pumpkin Custard

Wednesday

- Breakfast: Pear Nectar
- Lunch: Turnip and Leek Soup
- Dinner: Turkey and Vegetable Loaf
- Snack: Apple Ginger Tea

Thursday

- Breakfast: Watermelon Juice
- Lunch: Steamed Beet Greens
- Dinner: Chicken Tenderloins in Broth
- Snack: Oat Milk Latte

Friday

- Breakfast: Pumpkin Porridge
- Lunch: Braised Leeks
- Dinner: Grilled Turkey Breast
- Snack: Blueberry Oat Smoothie

Saturday

- Breakfast: Apple Ginger Tea
- Lunch: Stuffed Zucchini
- Dinner: Turkey and Sweet Potato Stew
- Snack: Pear Nectar

Sunday

- Breakfast: Banana Almond Smoothie
- Lunch: Roasted Root Vegetables
- Dinner: Oven-Roasted Turkey Breast
- Snack: Peach Smoothie

Week 4

Monday

- Breakfast: Watermelon Juice
- Lunch: Green Beans Almondine
- Dinner: Chicken Porridge
- Snack: Blueberry Oat Smoothie

Tuesday

- Breakfast: Pear Nectar
- Lunch: Celery Root Slaw
- Dinner: Turkey Apple Burgers
- Snack: Pumpkin Custard

Wednesday
- Breakfast: Coconut Rice Dessert
- Lunch: Steamed Artichokes
- Dinner: Chicken with Mashed Potatoes
- Snack: Apple Ginger Tea

Thursday
- Breakfast: Pumpkin Porridge
- Lunch: Squash and Apple Soup
- Dinner: Slow Cooker Chicken with Carrots
- Snack: Banana Almond Smoothie

Friday
- Breakfast: Peach Smoothie
- Lunch: Beetroot and Carrot Salad
- Dinner: Turkey Quinoa Pilaf
- Snack: Pear Nectar

Saturday
- Breakfast: Blueberry Oat Smoothie
- Lunch: Braised Leeks
- Dinner: Chicken Rice Paper Rolls
- Snack: Oat Milk Latte

Sunday
- Breakfast: Apple Ginger Tea
- Lunch: Herbed New Potatoes
- Dinner: Baked Turkey Meatloaf
- Snack: Watermelon Juice

Week 5

Monday
- Breakfast: Pear Nectar
- Lunch: Roasted Brussels Sprouts
- Dinner: Grilled Turkey Breast
- Snack: Blueberry Oat Smoothie

Tuesday
- Breakfast: Banana Almond Smoothie
- Lunch: Fennel and Apple Salad
- Dinner: Chicken and Vegetable Skewers
- Snack: Pumpkin Custard

Wednesday
- Breakfast: Watermelon Juice
- Lunch: Turnip and Leek Soup
- Dinner: Turkey and Zucchini Patties
- Snack: Oat Milk Latte

Thursday

- Breakfast: Pumpkin Porridge
- Lunch: Steamed Beet Greens
- Dinner: Chicken Tenderloins in Broth
- Snack: Pear Nectar

Friday

- Breakfast: Coconut Rice Dessert
- Lunch: Squash and Apple Soup
- Dinner: Slow Cooker Chicken with Carrots
- Snack: Blueberry Oat Smoothie

Saturday

- Breakfast: Apple Ginger Tea
- Lunch: Stuffed Zucchini
- Dinner: Turkey Quinoa Pilaf
- Snack: Banana Almond Smoothie

Sunday

- Breakfast: Peach Smoothie
- Lunch: Green Beans Almondine
- Dinner: Oven-Roasted Turkey Breast
- Snack: Pear Nectar

Week 6

Monday

- Breakfast: Blueberry Oat Smoothie
- Lunch: Steamed Beet Greens
- Dinner: Baked Parsnips
- Snack: Watermelon Juice

Tuesday

- Breakfast: Peach Smoothie
- Lunch: Green Beans Almondine
- Dinner: Chicken and Pear Salad
- Snack: Banana Almond Smoothie

Wednesday

- Breakfast: Coconut Rice Dessert
- Lunch: Fennel and Apple Salad
- Dinner: Turkey Spinach Quiche
- Snack: Pear Nectar

Thursday

- Breakfast: Apple Ginger Tea
- Lunch: Turnip and Leek Soup
- Dinner: Baked Chicken with Herbs
- Snack: Oat Milk Latte

Friday
- Breakfast: Banana Almond Smoothie
- Lunch: Celery Root Slaw
- Dinner: Turkey and Sweet Potato Stew
- Snack: Pumpkin Custard

Saturday
- Breakfast: Pear Nectar
- Lunch: Herbed New Potatoes
- Dinner: Chicken Tenderloins in Broth
- Snack: Watermelon Juice

Sunday
- Breakfast: Peach Smoothie
- Lunch: Steamed Artichokes
- Dinner: Grilled Turkey Breast
- Snack: Blueberry Oat Smoothie

Week 7

Monday
- Breakfast: Pumpkin Porridge
- Lunch: Beetroot and Carrot Salad
- Dinner: Turkey and Zucchini Patties
- Snack: Apple Ginger Tea

Tuesday
- Breakfast: Coconut Rice Dessert
- Lunch: Roasted Brussels Sprouts
- Dinner: Slow Cooker Chicken with Carrots
- Snack: Banana Almond Smoothie

Wednesday
- Breakfast: Pear Nectar
- Lunch: Braised Leeks
- Dinner: Chicken Porridge
- Snack: Oat Milk Latte

Thursday
- Breakfast: Peach Smoothie
- Lunch: Green Beans Almondine
- Dinner: Baked Turkey Meatloaf
- Snack: Watermelon Juice

Friday
- Breakfast: Blueberry Oat Smoothie
- Lunch: Fennel and Apple Salad
- Dinner: Turkey Quinoa Pilaf
- Snack: Apple Ginger Tea

Saturday

- Breakfast: Banana Almond Smoothie
- Lunch: Turnip and Leek Soup
- Dinner: Oven-Roasted Turkey Breast
- Snack: Pumpkin Custard

Sunday

- Breakfast: Pear Nectar
- Lunch: Steamed Beet Greens
- Dinner: Grilled Turkey Breast
- Snack: Blueberry Oat Smoothie

Week 8

Monday

- Breakfast: Coconut Rice Dessert
- Lunch: Squash and Apple Soup
- Dinner: Chicken and Vegetable Skewers
- Snack: Pear Nectar

Tuesday

- Breakfast: Pumpkin Porridge
- Lunch: Celery Root Slaw
- Dinner: Turkey Apple Burgers
- Snack: Watermelon Juice

Wednesday

- Breakfast: Apple Ginger Tea
- Lunch: Herbed New Potatoes
- Dinner: Chicken Pea Soup
- Snack: Blueberry Oat Smoothie

Thursday

- Breakfast: Peach Smoothie
- Lunch: Steamed Artichokes
- Dinner: Turkey and Vegetable Loaf
- Snack: Banana Almond Smoothie

Friday

- Breakfast: Blueberry Oat Smoothie
- Lunch: Roasted Root Vegetables
- Dinner: Chicken Rice Paper Rolls
- Snack: Apple Ginger Tea

Saturday

- Breakfast: Banana Almond Smoothie
- Lunch: Braised Leeks
- Dinner: Grilled Turkey Breast
- Snack: Pear Nectar

Sunday
- Breakfast: Coconut Rice Dessert
- Lunch: Green Beans Almondine
- Dinner: Slow Cooker Chicken with Carrots
- Snack: Pumpkin Custard

Week 9

Monday
- Breakfast: Pear Nectar
- Lunch: Beetroot and Carrot Salad
- Dinner: Turkey and Sweet Potato Stew
- Snack: Watermelon Juice

Tuesday
- Breakfast: Apple Ginger Tea
- Lunch: Turnip and Leek Soup
- Dinner: Baked Chicken with Herbs
- Snack: Blueberry Oat Smoothie

Wednesday
- Breakfast: Pumpkin Porridge
- Lunch: Celery Root Slaw
- Dinner: Chicken Tenderloins in Broth
- Snack: Banana Almond Smoothie

Thursday
- Breakfast: Peach Smoothie
- Lunch: Steamed Artichokes
- Dinner: Oven-Roasted Turkey Breast
- Snack: Pear Nectar

Friday
- Breakfast: Blueberry Oat Smoothie
- Lunch: Roasted Brussels Sprouts
- Dinner: Chicken and Pear Salad
- Snack: Apple Ginger Tea

Saturday
- Breakfast: Banana Almond Smoothie
- Lunch: Fennel and Apple Salad
- Dinner: Turkey Spinach Quiche
- Snack: Pumpkin Custard

Sunday
- Breakfast: Coconut Rice Dessert
- Lunch: Green Beans Almondine
- Dinner: Turkey Quinoa Pilaf
- Snack: Watermelon Juice

Week 10

Monday

- Breakfast: Pear Nectar
- Lunch: Braised Leeks
- Dinner: Chicken Porridge
- Snack: Blueberry Oat Smoothie

Tuesday

- Breakfast: Pumpkin Porridge
- Lunch: Squash and Apple Soup
- Dinner: Turkey and Zucchini Patties
- Snack: Apple Ginger Tea

Wednesday

- Breakfast: Coconut Rice Dessert
- Lunch: Celery Root Slaw
- Dinner: Slow Cooker Chicken with Carrots
- Snack: Banana Almond Smoothie

Thursday

- Breakfast: Peach Smoothie
- Lunch: Herbed New Potatoes
- Dinner: Chicken Pea Soup
- Snack: Pear Nectar

Friday

- Breakfast: Blueberry Oat Smoothie
- Lunch: Steamed Beet Greens
- Dinner: Turkey Apple Burgers
- Snack: Watermelon Juice

Saturday

- Breakfast: Banana Almond Smoothie
- Lunch: Turnip and Leek Soup
- Dinner: Grilled Turkey Breast
- Snack: Pumpkin Custard

Sunday

- Breakfast: Apple Ginger Tea
- Lunch: Roasted Root Vegetables
- Dinner: Baked Turkey Meatloaf
- Snack: Blueberry Oat Smoothie

WEEKLY MEAL PLANNER + WORKBOOK

	BREAKFAST	LUNCH	DINNER	SNACKS
MONDAY				
TUESDAY				
WEDNESDAY				
THURSDAY				
FRIDAY				
SATURDAY				
SUNDAY				

Reflect on your current symptoms. How severe are they and how do they impact your daily life?

WEEKLY MEAL PLANNER + WORKBOOK

	BREAKFAST	LUNCH	DINNER	SNACKS
MONDAY				
TUESDAY				
WEDNESDAY				
THURSDAY				
FRIDAY				
SATURDAY				
SUNDAY				

List three foods or beverages that you suspect might trigger discomfort or worsen your symptoms. How do you plan to avoid them?

WEEKLY MEAL PLANNER + WORKBOOK

	BREAKFAST	LUNCH	DINNER	SNACKS
MONDAY				
TUESDAY				
WEDNESDAY				
THURSDAY				
FRIDAY				
SATURDAY				
SUNDAY				

Consider your typical meal patterns before your ulcer diagnosis. What changes do you anticipate making to align with the peptic ulcer diet?

....

....

....

....

....

....

WEEKLY MEAL PLANNER + WORKBOOK

	BREAKFAST	LUNCH	DINNER	SNACKS
MONDAY				
TUESDAY				
WEDNESDAY				
THURSDAY				
FRIDAY				
SATURDAY				
SUNDAY				

Reflect on your hydration habits. How do you plan to ensure you're drinking enough fluids while managing ulcer symptoms?

WEEKLY MEAL PLANNER + WORKBOOK

	BREAKFAST	LUNCH	DINNER	SNACKS
MONDAY				
TUESDAY				
WEDNESDAY				
THURSDAY				
FRIDAY				
SATURDAY				
SUNDAY				

Identify any dietary habits or preferences that you believe might need to change to support your healing. Why are these changes important?

....

....

....

....

....

WEEKLY MEAL PLANNER + WORKBOOK

	BREAKFAST	LUNCH	DINNER	SNACKS
MONDAY				
TUESDAY				
WEDNESDAY				
THURSDAY				
FRIDAY				
SATURDAY				
SUNDAY				

What are your main concerns or challenges about starting the peptic ulcer diet? How do you plan to address these concerns?

WEEKLY MEAL PLANNER + WORKBOOK

	BREAKFAST	LUNCH	DINNER	SNACKS
MONDAY				
TUESDAY				
WEDNESDAY				
THURSDAY				
FRIDAY				
SATURDAY				
SUNDAY				

List three new foods or ingredients recommended for the peptic ulcer diet that you're willing to incorporate into your meals. What benefits do you expect from including these items?

....

....

....

....

....

....

WEEKLY MEAL PLANNER + WORKBOOK

	BREAKFAST	LUNCH	DINNER	SNACKS
MONDAY				
TUESDAY				
WEDNESDAY				
THURSDAY				
FRIDAY				
SATURDAY				
SUNDAY				

How do you plan to navigate social situations or dining out while adhering to the peptic ulcer diet?

....

....

....

....

....

WEEKLY MEAL PLANNER + WORKBOOK

	BREAKFAST	LUNCH	DINNER	SNACKS
MONDAY				
TUESDAY				
WEDNESDAY				
THURSDAY				
FRIDAY				
SATURDAY				
SUNDAY				

Consider your support system. How can family members or friends assist you in maintaining the peptic ulcer diet?

WEEKLY MEAL PLANNER + WORKBOOK

	BREAKFAST	LUNCH	DINNER	SNACKS
MONDAY				
TUESDAY				
WEDNESDAY				
THURSDAY				
FRIDAY				
SATURDAY				
SUNDAY				

What strategies will you use to track your food intake and monitor how your body responds to different foods on the peptic ulcer diet?

....

....

....

....

....

....

Scan the QR code below to get a surprise bonus!